How to Thrive in Professional Practice

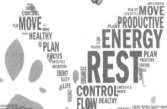

A SELF-CARE HANDBOOK

Other books you may be interested In:

Relationship-based Social Work with Adults
Edited by Heidi Dix, Sue Hollinrake and Jen Meade
ISBN 978-1-912096-27-5

Safeguarding Adults Together under the Care Act 2014: A Multi-agency Practice Guide
By Barbara Starns
ISBN 978-1-913063-25-2

Self-neglect: A Practical Approach to Risks and Strengths Assessment
By Shona Britten and Karen Whitby
ISBN 978-1-912096-86-2

The Social Worker's Guide to the Care Act, Second Edition
by Pete Feldon
ISBN 978-1-913453-05-3

Working with Family Carers
By Valerie Gant
ISBN 978-1-912096-978

Titles are also available in a range of electronic formats. To order please go to our website www.criticalpublishing.com or contact our distributor NBN International, 10 Thornbury Road, Plymouth PL6 7PP, telephone 01752 202301 or email orders@nbninternational.com

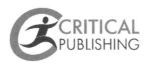

How to Thrive in Professional Practice

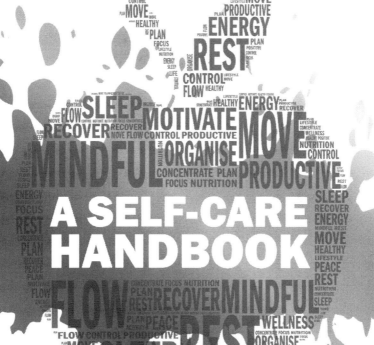

A SELF-CARE HANDBOOK

Stephen J Mordue, Lisa Watson and Steph Hunter

First published in 2020 by Critical Publishing Ltd

British Library Cataloguing in Publication Data
A CIP record for this book is available from the British Library

ISBN: 9781913063894

This book is also available in the following ebook formats:
MOBI ISBN: 9781913063900
EPUB ISBN: 9781913063917
Adobe ebook ISBN: 9781913063924

Cover design by Out of House
Text design by Greensplash Limited
Project Management by Newgen Publishing UK
Printed and bound in the UK by 4edge, Essex

Critical Publishing
3 Connaught Road
St Albans
AL3 5RX

www.criticalpublishing.com

Paper from responsible sources

Contents

Meet the authors

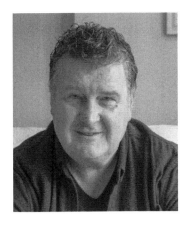

Stephen J Mordue

Stephen has 19 years' experience in social work, initially as a practitioner and team manager working with older people and for the last seven years as a lecturer in social work specialising in adult care and the Mental Capacity Act and Best Interests Assessment. He works at the University of Sunderland.

He found some self-care ideas more by chance than design as an avid runner and spiritual enquirer. He's a great fan of mindfulness and meditation as an 'easy to access', 'no gear required' approach to well-being. Having spent most of his life being completely disorganised he was told about David Allen's 'Getting Things Done' methodology and so his new life began!

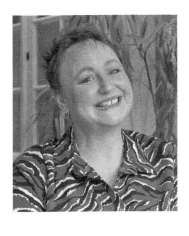

Lisa Watson

Lisa has over 25 years' experience of working in health and social care settings, ranging from occupational therapy to social work. She graduated as a mature student from Sunderland University with BA (Hons) Social Work in 2008.

Following job demands and burnout, she took a career break for two years and set up a holistic business, undertaking training in mindfulness and life coaching. Spiritual in her approach to life and practice, Lisa resumed social work and passionately teaches others about the importance of professional self-care. Lisa lives in Sunderland and in her spare time enjoys reading, music and all things spiritual.

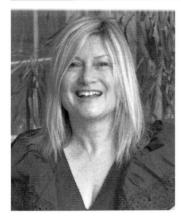

Steph Hunter

Steph has been a social worker for 23 years. During her career, she has worked in Cafcass, children and families, and substance misuse. The main focus of her career has been children's mental health and she managed an award-winning mental health service for looked after children and adopted children for over a decade. This won three national awards and three regional NHS awards. From 2015 to 2019 Steph was a Senior Lecturer at Sunderland University, where she met Stephen and valued his self-care ideas.

Her interest in self-care began when she managed the mental health team. Some of the developments she was involved in included a lunchtime running club and shared lunches with key partners.

Steph is particularly passionate about developing self-care for those at risk of secondary trauma, including foster carers and adoptive parents. Juggling the rigours of parenthood and work and study, she has learned the importance of caring for your own physical and emotional well-being for herself. She enjoys swimming, reading, travel and developing approaches to help children and families. One of her passions is being outdoors and she can usually be found at a beach at the weekend!

Steph has published in relation to adoption, looked after children, austerity and parenting, and has frequently spoken on the radio in relation to her areas of interest.

Acknowledgements

STEPHEN

I wouldn't have even thought about the things in this book if it hadn't been for my good friend Pete Wright showing me his 'Getting Things Done' spreadsheet and telling me about David Allen and the art of stress-free productivity. For that lightbulb moment, and his friendship, I will be forever in his debt.

Thanks to Gareth Clegg for being a constant source of inspiration from our first moments of friendship at age 12 and throughout my life. Though miles and time separate us, you are always there. Things that fit endure.

A huge thank you to the people I work with who have indulged me by letting me introduce the ideas contained in this book to the University of Sunderland's social work students. Thanks to the students who have endured my faltering explanation of all manner of things relating to self-care and productivity as I figured out how to say what I wanted to say. And a big thank you to Anna Short for sorting out my Self-care Triangle graphic!

And, without doubt, thanks to Christine, Jonathan and Luke for their unfathomable love that sustains me.

I dedicate my words written on these pages to my mam and dad who have always believed in me.

LISA

Some people have come into my life and made it great, others have made it great once they have left. I look to the blessings and lessons from every one of you, for they have made me who I am today.

Stephen Holmes and Lois Woods encouraged me to go to university and, in doing so, sowed the seeds of my social work career. I am truly thankful to you both as it started me on this amazing journey of self-discovery.

I give thanks to Stephen Mordue for agreeing to collaborate with me on a totally different project that led to interesting discussions around social work and self-care. This in turn snowballed into the idea of writing a book about professional self-care and hey, we did it – world domination next!

Finally, to quote Terri Guillemets, '*I love my mother as trees love water and sunshine, she helps me grow, prosper and reach great heights.*'

My 'mam' has been the single most loyal and consistent figure in my life. Unconditional love that knows no bounds. Guidance, wisdom and the same wicked humour has helped illuminate my way in life during times when I could not always see the way ahead. No words can ever truly reflect what you mean to me and I hope this book makes you proud, not just of me, but of you, for being 'you'.

STEPH

How lovely to get an opportunity to write in a book and then thank those who have supported you. It feels a little Oscar-like ... I can dream!

Thank you to Peter Twiss, my teacher at Kelloe Primary School who printed my first stories when I was at school and supported me. Thank you to Peter Raymond, my social studies teacher at Gilesgate School, who bought me chocolate when I stopped truanting. Thank you to my dad and brother, no longer with me but I feel they believed in me.

I was able to be part of this book possibly because I asked Stephen regularly if I could contribute while we passed on the stairs at university when I lectured there too. I also genuinely believe in self-care.

Thanks to Bev and Jo, psychiatrist friends, who responded to my many messages as I shared concern about my own self-care, and writing late at night! Thanks to Rachael Woodley, who is a self-care star and is one of the most encouraging people I know in spite of adversity herself.

Thanks to my boyfriend as he never likes to be left out and would seek a drum roll if pages were audio transcribed! He did divert me from this book at times but supported more than hindered.

Last but not least, thank you to my daughters Grace and Tilly, who showed me love and really are the reason I do everything. Thanks for reading.

'Begin with the end in mind.'

Stephen R Covey, *The 7 Habits of Highly Effective People*

Introduction: the reality of self-care

Stephen, Lisa and Steph

LET US BEGIN...

We have all got a unique story because we are all unique. The three of us writing this book all have our own tales to tell, and you will have yours. Your life has brought you to this point, so well done for getting here. At various points during your life you will, I'm sure, have tried very hard to do things. Sometimes you will have succeeded at your endeavours and sometimes, like us, you will have failed. Occasionally spectacularly. Such is life.

Self-care is like life. We try, we fail and we try again. The self-care prescription you require is unique to you. You will need bits of everything we talk about in these pages but in a unique balance that is all yours. Experimentation is key.

This book comes with a guarantee. All of the ideas that are in here have been tried and tested by one or all of us. We come to you as people who have given things a go and have generally ended up a little better off as a consequence. Small steps lead to big changes. You might read that phrase a few times in the coming pages. You have been warned. Self-care is not about getting it right all of the time. It's about getting it right as much as you can, realising you have neglected to get it right for a while, and knowing where to go back to in order to reengage with it. For engage with it we must.

For years on and off, my path and the paths of Lisa and Steph have kept intersecting. Snippets of conversations in corridors. Years of not seeing each other as our paths developed. During these snatched conversations there were nuggets of information behind the 'How are you?' 'Fine' type conversations that might have hinted that at times things were not fine. Lisa and I knew each other as practitioners in older people's services. I stayed and she left to go off into children and families social work, but we still bumped into each other occasionally. I knew Steph because she hosted student placements for us and then ended up working at the same university. Over time, the conversations developed and through a chance Facebook exchange Lisa and I started talking about meditation. We met for a coffee and discovered that our unique journeys had, as it turns out, a lot of commonality. There were stories of long hours, stressful cases, too much wine and too much comfort eating. The other common thread was that we were both trying to mitigate these things. Me, largely through exercise and Lisa, through holistic therapy.

What was clear was that there was more to what we were trying to do than mere chance. The stars had aligned (Lisa will like that line!) and we were up and running on a journey of discovery to find out just what lay behind our attempts to care for ourselves and what was hindering us. We hoped we might actually find out what would help us. What was the science behind sleep, what was the research about nutrition, and was there really something to mindfulness or was it just some hippy hangover from the sixties?

We started delivering self-care sessions to students and then to practitioners. What we discovered was that everyone, to one degree or another, was involved in the same struggle. Trying to cope with the emotional labour of social work or being a student. Trying to figure out how to explore feelings. Trying to figure out how to get things done and control the chaotic world. Trying to balance everything. Trying to fit everything in. Knowing that there must be a better way but not knowing what that better way might look like. '*If what you are doing isn't working then maybe it's time to do something different*', someone once said to me.

We live in an 'information overload' society so we knew all the relevant information was out there. What wasn't there in people's heads was the underpinning theory and science that said '*do this because we know it works*'. So, people were often cynical. '*How can going for a walk help?!*' '*How can focusing on my breathing make the slightest bit of difference?!*' What was also missing was people feeling ok about giving themselves permission to look after themselves. People could easily trot out phrases like '*I know! If I don't look after myself how can I look after others*', but they weren't heeding this advice, so stress and burnout were, and still are, rife. The research and people leaving the profession confirm this.

Hopefully this book is an adventure into the depths of what actually works in regard to self-care and why it works. The advice is not about running marathons, it's about the benefits of what is really only a small amount of regular exercise that gets you a little breathless. It's not about dieting so you are in a size 8 dress or have a 30-inch waist. It's about how what you eat influences your emotions and therefore your productivity. It's not about reaching the dizzy heights of a zen-like state when attempting meditation, but is about how small steps into mindfulness and meditation can influence how you emotionally respond to events around you. Mostly this book is about what we can do to help ourselves to have the best lives we can have, by being the best versions of ourselves we can be. Not perfect but rather living in a way that is productive and helpful to us and to those around us. Keeping ourselves in order so that we cope with the chaos out there.

We are not perfect and don't always get things right or even heed our own advice. We have all been on a journey to get to this point and there is more journey in front of us. We know what it's like to struggle so we thought it might be useful to share a little of our stories about what led us to contemplate self-care ideas before we get started.

Lisa's Storm to Calm

Thank you, Stephen, and yes, I loved that line about the stars aligning because it's so true, the stars were aligned!

I think it is important for us to share our story because it will help others to know we really do understand what it's like to crash and burn and have to get back up only to crash and burn again. Let's see if any of these phrases are familiar: professional stress, end of my tether, life falling apart, hate work, overworked, undervalued, stood at a crossroads in life, stuck, need to change but don't know how, depressed and tired?

It's not that long ago I was feeling most of these, but the thought of moving out of my comfort zone by making the desired changes was scary. It was this fear that kept me stuck on the treadmill of monotony, anxiety and boredom for longer than I should have been, resulting in my eventual total crash and burn that required a career break.

Truthfully, I just felt useless. Work made me constantly anxious, longing for the weekend but fearing not being at work. My overactive imagination would have me dealing with all kinds of crises come Monday morning. Friday would arrive like a long-lost relative, but I would be too tense to start to unwind. As a social worker, conditioned to reflect upon my practice, I thought this meant the need to constantly replay conversations in my head. Pondering what I could have done differently when that family member was screaming at me down the telephone and was making me shake with anxiety. Did feeling anxious make me come across as antagonistic rather than empathic? Over and over I'd replay the same scenario, thinking, thinking and thinking what I could have done differently.

On Saturday I'd spend all day thanking the heavens above I wasn't at work. On Sunday morning I would be hit with the realisation that *'tomorrow is Monday and I'm back to work'*. I would spend the rest of Sunday worrying about worst-case scenarios, imagining how every single one of my cases was bound to have 'kicked off' over the weekend and how goodness knows how many emails would be waiting for me as soon as I logged into the work PC. Monday morning was boooom! Rush hour traffic was usually navigated through a sea of tears and the much longed-for journey home was often undertaken in the same saltwater haze.

Yet, every Monday morning things were never as bad as my imagination would have had me believe. The really sad thing is, I had not had any relaxation all weekend due to unnecessary worry. I would arrive at work on a Monday morning already in a heightened state of stress, which would be exacerbated as the week progressed. I was stuck in this cycle of constantly being at work. When I was not physically at work, I was mentally and emotionally at work. Every second of every day, that's where I was. Something had to give, and I was given the opportunity to leave the profession I loved but had grown to despise. Social work and I had officially separated and filed for divorce.

So I set up my own holistic business, and trained in life coaching and mindfulness. While this took me down a road that ended up being a dead end, it offered me the opportunity of time and space to learn to reconnect with the person I am. What I came to realise is that social work, at that time, had stripped me of my identity, my sense of humour and who I was as an individual. This time and distance allowed to me to come to terms with the fact that social work is an extremely difficult and challenging profession. Yeah, I know, who knew eh? I'm back in practice again now.

I suppose I had always believed myself to be saving starfish. You know the story by Loren Eiseley (1979) where the little boy on a beach throws starfish back into the sea? He is asked by an adult why he is doing that as there are too many starfish stranded on the beach to make a difference. He responds by telling the adult he had made a difference to the one starfish he had just thrown back into the sea. For all my good intentions and goodwill, I was never going to fix the world. I was never going to 'save' everyone because no one can.

I hope with all my heart that even the smallest amount of truth of what is within this book resonates with you and that it may help you in your moment of Storm to reach a place of Calm.

Steph's story

Think in the morning. Act in the noon. Eat in the evening. Sleep in the night.

(William Blake)

When I sit and reflect on how long I have worked in social work, I think about how in my work with young people I have encountered some very sad cases over the years. That has sometimes made me question why I do the work I do. I have always struggled with the idea of how little social justice and what unequal starting points some people have in life, particularly in some of the vulnerable groups we work with. Despite this, I somehow find the strength to carry on, as I know how much my work means to me and, if I am honest, some of the best, most rewarding experiences in my life have been work related.

Buddhism helps me to see the world around me in a more positive light, and did so especially when my only brother died suddenly and tragically in 2018. He was the same age I am now, and his passing brings home to me how we are all on a journey in relation to self-care and just how important this is for each of us.

During my early social work career, I developed the healthy habit of sticking to core working hours, went to the gym close to my office, ate well and ensured I took my lunch breaks when I could. Leadership is what makes the difference. I always rate managers who set good examples and know the value of lunch breaks! They develop cultures in which micromanagement is discouraged and innovation is welcomed. I worked in the Children and Family Court Advisory and Support Service (Cafcass) until 2002. The culture at the time was unique to the warm but small team. It involved mid-morning coffee breaks and afternoon tea, and a shared garden was developed by a green-fingered colleague which allowed a relaxed approach to us sharing concerns about families, brainstorming and generally being emotionally available to each other as a means of managing risk issues. We also learned about each other's families and personal interests, so we got to know each other really well and were able to tell when one of us was struggling. This was great care in action. This type of team helps you deal with the difficult aspects of the work we do, like the day a mother screamed at me about how much she hated my voice. I still remember consciously listening to my own voice as I spoke to see if she had a point!

I try and enjoy a short walk during my lunch break, like Stephen, as I know this helps me return to my afternoon work feeling refreshed and focused. It was invaluable during my days of trying to juggle social work with an interest in performing arts when I ended up as an extra in a film. It was a very interesting time, juggling filming during the day with nocturnal report writing. Not the best in terms of self-care. Sadly, due to my dedication to social work and knowing I could not miss presenting a case in court, I had to forgo the chance to drive a Ferrari booked for the day when Patsy Kensit (who was the real star) was ill.

Over the years, despite my best of intentions, I'm afraid my healthy habits have slipped. I have a real sweet tooth so I'm always after my sugar boost. It doesn't help that I simply love baking cakes or scones for the team. But taking care of others, often to the detriment of myself, can take its toll. I push myself to be there for others, even when I know I am feeling tired. The body tells us when it needs to rest, if only we'd listen! I need to listen more! I've learned so much on the journey to help write this book and hope you take away some of the points that really resonate with you and hopefully help 'you' to take care of 'you'!

Stephen's story – the self-medication cycle

I've been quite lucky that over the years I have done many things by chance rather than design that have contributed to being in general good health and well-being. As you'll find out later in the book, I wasn't a fan of exercise at school, but as a young adult I found a great passion for running, weight training and squash, all of which helped mitigate my other passion, food. I do like to eat. Although again, by chance, I do enjoy for the most part quite healthy food. I just enjoy a lot of it!

I was brought up going to church so was conscious of the benefits of quiet contemplation and as a child and teenager, in a pre-computer game era, hanging out with friends was largely an outdoor pursuit. I carried this love of the outdoors with me throughout my adult life and, as we know, being outside is good for you. I have translated my faith as a younger person into adult enquiry about mindfulness and meditation as there are many parallels between those pursuits and the prayer that people of faith engage in.

I hadn't really had much cause to consider self-care as I was engaging in self-care activities without really realising I was. But then as a social worker things took a bit of a turn. I found myself struggling with difficult cases and found it difficult to keep myself organised. I got into the habit of leaving things until the last minute. I hit that dangerous place most of us get to where we think we know what we're doing. In reality, especially in a profession like social work, you never completely know what you are doing and always need to be learning and developing. I lost focus and felt as though I was always trying to keep up. I did keep up, nothing went wrong, everything got done, but it was all done in quite a chaotic way. This was exacerbated when I became a manager. There's an assumption that because you are good at one thing, you will be good at another, and while I think I did a fine job as a manager, it came at a cost. I relate to what Lisa was saying above when she talked about thinking about work all the time.

My solution was to drink wine. Every night. This was the only way I could get to sleep. This inevitably led to a hangover the next day, which meant that I drank copious amounts of coffee. I was an expert in the caffeine crash. Drinking so much wine and coffee made me feel dreadful, but all was well as I found a solution. Over-the-counter medication in the form of codeine took away the dreadful stomach pains and headaches I was feeling in the early afternoon and gave me a relaxed feeling. Codeine is an opiate so is very addictive. It also makes you constipated, and coffee, as you may know, agitates the bowel and can help you go to the toilet. Can you imagine! Internal uproar, which led to feeling even more lousy, which meant the cycle of alcohol, caffeine and codeine to try and feel better started again. A conversation with a friend who is a doctor alerted me to the harm codeine was doing to me when taken regularly and I stopped immediately.

I look back on that period of time now, probably a period of around six months, and reflect on how dreadful I felt day in, day out. That cycle was driven by stress and by not knowing how to manage the stress I was feeling in a positive way. I chose a negative route. Ultimately, choosing a negative route makes you feel worse in the long run. The difficulty is that negative routes are often easier. It takes commitment to look after yourself properly and do the right thing for your body and mind. It's all about developing healthy habits.

THRIVING IN PROFESSIONAL PRACTICE

Enough about us. Let's get started. We have found out so much on our various journeys that we want to share with you. Small steps really do make a big difference. I'd suggest you grab yourself a pen and a notebook because I think you'll find it really useful to make notes as you go and jot down your responses to some of the questions we will pose for you. Writing things down helps to consolidate ideas and makes action more likely. Books are tools so I give you permission to write in the margins and underline things and put big asterisks against the bits you want to find again. And if you want to break the spine of the book so you can lay it flat, go on, do it.

Let's go.

REFERENCE

Eiseley, Loren (1979) *The Star Thrower.* New York: Harvest.

1 Self-care: the fundamental principles

Stephen

THE CONTEXT

The modern world is a stressful place. Our physical and mental attributes that evolved many centuries ago were designed to deal with a very different world to the one we find ourselves in today. The Industrial Revolution saw the creation of cities and factories and a working day that never needed to stop. Electricity meant the lights were always on and if the lights were always on then the people could always be working and the owners of the 'means of production', the bourgeoisie, as Marx named them, could always be earning more money. No longer were we subject to the coming and going of day and night and the turning of the seasons, but rather we were chained to the wheel of capitalism. Then capitalism sold us the dream. The architects of advertising, the manufacturers of consumerism, told us that if we were working hard we could afford to buy all manner of things and in buying all manner of things we could be transformed into the best version of ourselves by surrounding ourselves with stuff that shows how successful we are. I'd argue that we are currently seeing a backlash against this with many people turning inward to find fulfilment internally through nutrition, meditation and minimalist lifestyles. Yet we still live, work and play in the world as it is.

The problem is that once you are on the treadmill it is hard to get off. The bills need to be paid; the mortgage needs to be covered. The repayments for the car need to be found so that you can get to the job that helps you pay for it. In all of that, somewhere, despite the efforts of 1960s counterculture, we lost ourselves. Our identity has become bound up in the things we have rather than the people we are. What we are has become more important than who we are. The first question we always ask at a party is '*What do you do?*' Invariably we respond by telling the person what we do for a paid job. You probably say, '*I'm a social worker*'. Or maybe you don't! We could respond differently, '*I'm an adventurer at the boundaries of the capacity of my mind and body.*' But we don't. And there it is, we are defined, with all of the baggage that goes with the label and nothing about who we are, of which 'social worker' is merely one part.

James et al (2019) say 'social worker' *is* very much who you are and not what you are, alluding to the pervasive, life-absorbing nature of the role. We bring ourselves and everything we are to the job. That means being professional, empathetic, sympathetic, driven, always there for people, sacrificing, giving, going the extra mile and taking one for the team. The problem is that underneath all of that giving of self we run the risk of slowly disappearing. When this happens, we slowly detach ourselves from the very people we came into the job to support. The literature on this subject has defined this *compassion fatigue'.* The problems and distress that you hear about and uncover become just part of the job and the risk is that you simply start to process people. The stories feel familiar, so everyone gets the same response. Such an approach, though, is not satisfying and merely compounds the problem, and compassion fatigue leads to burnout which leads to presenteeism. You are at work, but you are not really at work. You are there physically going through the motions but mentally you are detached, distant. If this continues you will burn out. Peterson (2018, p 60) makes the sobering point that not only can a lack of self-care have implications for you, but also *'mistreatment of yourself can have catastrophic effects on others'*. Failure to take steps to care for yourself and be able to adequately discharge your professional responsibilities could have an impact on you, the people who are 'in your care' and your family, as a direct consequence of your poor physical and mental health.

WHO ARE SOCIAL WORKERS AND WHERE IS SOCIAL WORK HAPPENING?

Social workers undoubtedly come from a range of backgrounds and the social work role is to support a diverse range of people. The role is steeped in ambiguity and uncertainty as individuals, including you, are unique. We are right in among the 'messy stuff' as James et al (2019) put it. Yet despite this, social work, in local authorities at least, is organised and managed in what can be an inflexible, bureaucratic, hierarchical structure (Gibson, 2017). In contrast to this lack of flexibility, social work exists in a constantly changing environment, influenced by emerging theoretical ideas, the political ideology of the day and the nature of the 'person-facing' work it undertakes. It is often driven by crisis management and social problems (Deacon, 2017; Griffiths, 2017). These two realities are at odds with each other. Handy (1999) describes a 'role' culture that is reflective of the culture in local authorities. In a 'role' culture there are clear policies and guidelines, clear structures and clear lines of accountability. Role cultures are suitable in organisations that are not subject to frequent change and where there is predictability. While this may well have been the case for local authorities many years ago, it is not the case now. What is now required is openness and responsiveness rather than the traditional bureaucratic hierarchy (Hughes and Wearing, 2017). Where there is a mismatch like this between the organisational structure and culture and the needs of the wider environment in which people are asked to operate, there is a risk that employees may not thrive and may well experience stress due to competing internal and external demands. In terms of well-being, such an organisation may well have procedural responses to people's well-being once they are unwell rather than an individualised, person-centred approach that tries to mitigate the problem before it occurs.

THE SOCIAL WORKER 'TYPE'

Luetchford (2015) observes that social workers are a particular 'type'. He notes that in his time as a manager he has had to send staff home who were clearly unwell but had come to work out of a sense of duty. This may well be as a consequence of one of the very things that attracts people to social work practice: the desire to not leave people unassisted or excluded. He alludes to the fact that social workers find it hard to say '*no*' and states that mechanisms to challenge employers are few. There is a risk here that social workers continue to accept unrealistic levels of stress as the norm and this makes them unwell. Sickness presenteeism (being at work when unwell, physically or mentally) can have both an impact on the quality of the work done by the employee and an obvious negative health consequence. Sickness absence, on the other hand, can be a time for physical and psychological recovery. The risk, however, extrapolating the idea that people are reluctant to be absent from work, is that people may not engage in dialogue about self-care as they may see this as weakness and not want to be perceived as 'struggling' with workload (Skagen and Collins, 2016).

THE DEMANDS OF THE WORKPLACE

Marc and Osvat (2013) report that organisational challenges are predominantly reported as being the greatest source of stress, noting, for example, deadlines, hierarchies, insufficient time, high caseloads, excessive bureaucracy, insufficient resources and poor management as stressors. Interestingly, respondents in their research cite solutions to the problem of stress as being outside of the workplace – for example, movement therapy, family support, conversations with colleagues and friends, walks and unplanned vacations. Predominantly, people seem to construct the problem *in the workplace* yet solve it *outside of the workplace*. This seems to suggest that employees do not see their employers as having a role in mitigating the risks of work-related stress. This is reflective of the neoliberal agenda that seeks to place self-governance outside of the state and individualise responsibility for well-being (Crawshaw, 2012). But maybe this is the way it is. There is an inherent reality in this about how much an employer can actually do when self-care does indeed need to be initiated at an individual level. The answer is possibly a two-pronged attack, with employers raising awareness of self-care and mitigating some of the stressors as far as is possible, while people commit to taking personal responsibility for being organised, and for their own nutrition, exercise and sleep.

REFLECTIVE TASK

What type of social worker are you?
What is the culture of the organisation you work in?
What are the workplace demands that create stress for you?
What do you do at work to mitigate the stress you feel?
What do you do outside of work to mitigate the stress you feel?

LEADERSHIP

Sánchez-Moreno et al (2015) report that, alongside other factors, structures within social work organisations and the organisational environment, lack of clarity in role and lack of supervision are determinants in relation to burnout. This seems to be reflective of the tension between organisational culture and the requirements of the task environment. In order to adequately explore the impact of the workplace, a critical perspective is required which will ensure an understanding that reflects the employee's position so that real attempts can be made to find solutions.

Leadership style is important in achieving an understanding of the employee's position. Echoing the practice development ethos of person-centredness, a leader should make decisions in collaboration, and motivate and lead by example. This ensures a sharing of decision-making power and ultimately a sharing of responsibility (Heyns et al, 2017). In relation to well-being this is essential as many of the solutions to promoting well-being can be counter-intuitive or go against organisational culture. Levitin (2015) observes that '*the companies that are winning the productivity battle are those that allow their employees productivity hours, naps, a chance for exercise, and a calm, tranquil, orderly environment in which to do their work*' (Levitin, 2015, p 307). This goes against the 'lunch at your desk' philosophy that permeates many social work teams. Davidson (2015) reported in *The Telegraph* research from BUPA that stated that two thirds of British workers are not even able to stop for 20 minutes for lunch. This has an impact on well-being and productivity as we shall see later. Ultimately, self-care needs to be a joint responsibility.

A WORD OF CAUTION

I want to proceed with caution here but need to state clearly what I have already alluded to. It is not appropriate to place the onus to solve all of social work's ills on the individual. There are clearly ideological, funding and organisational issues at play that are also worthy of investigation and transformation. It is apparent that social care resources and social work practice are underfunded, and it is felt by many that caseloads are too high. My concern, however, is that social work has created and is perpetuating a narrative that says that front-line social workers can do nothing about this. This is not true. There is a need to keep making our voices heard through our regulator and through the ballot box, but in the meantime, how do we keep ourselves well? That is the purpose of this book. We do not propose that the tools and ideas we present are a panacea for all of the problems in the profession but we do strongly feel that they have the potential to transform how we feel about ourselves and the work we do so that we can maintain a level of well-being.

Karen Healy (2014), drawing on Foucault's writings on power, is clear. Power is everywhere, is productive, and is exercised rather than possessed. This means the power to change the 'whole' position we find ourselves in can be exercised through the power we find in ourselves to change and think differently. She talks about power needing to be analysed from the bottom up. Where is your power? It is unlikely you can change the onslaught of caseloads, court of protection reports and multi-disciplinary meetings, in the short term at least. But maybe you change how you approach them, how you plan for them and what you do in terms of your self-care to ensure you are as ready for them, physically, mentally and emotionally, as you can be.

WE ARE A PART OF THE WHOLE

The reality is we are a part of the organisation in which the social work we do takes place. Being part of it and knowing how it functions is an important aspect in what we need to do. Hughes and Wearing (2017, p 80) observe that social workers need to be '*competent, strategic and ethical organisational operators*', so therefore need to be an active part of the organisation and understand it. I feel that sometimes some social workers take up an anti-organisation stance. The problem with this is that it creates an environment in which hostility can breed. While conflict, in the broadest terms, is an inevitable part of any relationship, it should drive consensus rather than produce a stand-off. Having a negative attitude to work saps your psychological well-being, generates stress and demotivates. This then restricts your productivity. Netting et al (1993, p 123) state that '*social workers with little or no idea of how organisations operate, or how they are influenced and changed by both outside and inside are likely to be severely limited in their effectiveness*'. Or, put simply, you need to know how to work as part of the system with all of its flaws in order to be productive. You need to work with it and challenge it to change rather than be in conflict with it.

EMOTIONAL LABOUR

The emotional labour that social work is comes with inevitable tensions. Organisational strategies and the reality of limited resources often feel in stark contrast to social work values and this can have a strong demotivating effect. It seems to be a fact that there has to be some level of acceptance of the bureaucracy that is inevitable in large organisations. We have seen above that the things social workers report as being stressful are the bureaucratic elements. Hughes and Wearing (2017) describe the stress in organisations as resulting from the intensification of work and I'm sure that anyone working in social work can attest to this. Does this intensification come from the face-to-face work or from the paperwork? The answer I hear most is it is the latter.

Providing professional social work support in such an environment can still remain a significantly rewarding profession. It does involve dealing with, and often trying to change, people's emotional responses to situations that are frequently born out of trauma. Such work clearly does come at an emotional cost to the practitioner (Adams et al, 2006). This emotional component can easily manifest itself as stress, which can be acute (short term) or chronic (long term). The impact of the emotional nature of the role is compounded by workplace demands like case conferences, report writing and tight deadlines as well as stressors of everyday personal life that can seriously impact on the practitioner's overall well-being and performance (Grant et al, 2014). There is a relationship between work life and personal life.

The focus on the well-being of you as a practitioner is important given the emotional cost of practice (Adams et al, 2006). This cost has the potential for both short-term and long-term stress leading to illness, absence from work and people leaving the profession. The Health and Care Professions Council (2016) reported an increase in turnover of social work staff from 12 per cent in 2014 to 16 per cent in 2016 with vacancy rates up from 3 per cent to 11 per cent in the same period. As Sánchez-Moreno et al (2015) point out, social workers are an 'at risk' group when it comes to work-based stress as a consequence of the complex nature of their role and exposure to the distress they often witness.

STRESS

Professional work is demanding, and stress is not in essence wholly negative. *The Guardian* (2019) has recently reported that research shows that stress can improve resilience. When we encounter some pressure, we are motivated to meet the challenge of the circumstances in front of us. It is when we become overwhelmed and our usual coping strategies have run out that we become stressed and ultimately distressed. This has significant connotations for our emotional, mental and physical well-being (Grant and Kinman, 2014) as it would appear the avoidance of stress is also not wholly positive and can lead to inertia. A balance is required. Some of the problems associated with stress can be mitigated through positive self-care and indeed resilience is felt to be something that can be developed and can positively influence physical and mental health (Stacey et al, 2017).

While the people we work for do have a responsibility for our well-being, self-management is also key. Grafton and Coyne (2012) tell us that what does us harm is not the stress itself but our response to it. So, we have to take some responsibility for ourselves. Often in the caring professions we are so busy helping others that we neglect self-care and then are not able to fully engage in the day (Bent-Goodley, 2018). We need to step back and think about what we are doing to ourselves and consider seriously how better to care for ourselves and encourage an '*attitude and practice of having compassion for oneself*' (Iacono, 2017, p 454) rather than saving it all for others.

A BALANCED LIFE

It can be difficult when feeling stressed to compartmentalise the impact of work-based stress and personal life stress to figure out where the stressor lies, as each can have an impact on the other. That's why what we propose in this book is a whole-life approach to well-being and self-care. The separation of 'work' and 'life' is socially constructed and unhelpful in terms of well-being. As Mihaly Csikszentmihalyi states:

> *Once we realize that the boundaries between work and play are artificial, we can take matters in hand and begin the difficult task of making life more liveable.*
>
> (Csikszentmihalyi, 2000, p 190)

It is true that in order to establish and maintain well-being we need balance. As you will see through this book, how we balance the physical, mental and spiritual aspects of our life is important as they all interact and have an impact on each other. To try to separate these aspects into things that happen during 'work' and things that happen during 'life' is artificial and misses the point of how connected all of the things in our lives are. The term work–life balance is a fairly recent one. It didn't really appear in our vocabulary until the 1980s and coincided with an increase in women joining the workforce in large numbers. Work–life balance was then about how women balanced their traditional role in the home with their new role at work. It took men a little longer to catch on to this idea (it usually does!) and it wasn't until the 1990s that men started talking in these terms. A study of the top 100 newspapers and magazines showed a paltry 32 mentions between 1986 and 1996, rising to a high of 1,674 mentions in 2007. The idea had become firmly rooted in our language (Keller and Papasan, 2014), but it is not a wholly helpful concept.

The problem with the concept of work–life balance is it creates an artificial separation and promotes a psychology of work being the thing to get done and out of the way so that you can get at this thing called 'life'. This leads to a resentment of work and a desire to not be there. But, as Cannon (2018) says, what we do as a job is a significant part of our lives and provides a sense of achievement, success and pride. It gives us status socially and economically and can promote our self-esteem. The job is more than just a job for lots of us and that is particularly true for social workers and other 'people' professions. James et al (2019, p 44) make this notable point, saying that if you find that being a social worker '*stops for you at 5.30 p.m., then you need to have a good old social work self-reflection session and if it still stops for you at 5.30 p.m., then perhaps it never started at 9 a.m. in the first place*'. What I don't feel they are saying here is that you should be writing up case notes or court reports at 10pm every night or have a life dominated by work tasks. What they are saying, I'd suggest, is that a profession such as social work is all consuming. It is, as mentioned earlier, *who* you are not *what* you are. This means you may well find yourself thinking about, reading about and possibly doing social work outside of the usual office hours. This is fine – but it has to be a healthy balance and not to the detriment of your overall well-being. But, and here's the point, a well-managed professional life and a well-managed personal life can exist harmoniously.

Why not think about a balanced life differently? I look at life like this. There are some things I do that I get paid for. There are some things I do that I don't get paid for but still do because I enjoy doing them, and there are things I do to recover from the 'doing'. These three aspects are all important and it is these three aspects I need to balance. I need to get paid for some things as I live in a society where we exchange our time for money and money for things we need. I also do things I don't get paid for that are about self-development or self-worth, or to support others. I then have to recover from doing all of that. The idea is to live a balanced life not to balance work and life *with* each other, as what often happens is that they are balanced *against* each other. When you are working with a family and achieve a great outcome, or when you finish that difficult report you had to write, and you are proud of what you have done – does that not feel like 'life'? When you are at home and you are doing the ironing, or folding the socks, does that not feel like work? The elements of life that we call 'work' exist whether we are in the office or at home and the elements of life that we call 'life', those joyous, pleasurable moments of an outcome achieved or a task complete, exist both in the office and in the home. Or they should.

REFLECTIVE TASK

- What do you do that you get paid for?
- What do you enjoy about what you get paid for?
- What do you not enjoy about what you get paid for?
- What do you do that you don't get paid for?

- What do you enjoy about what you do that you don't get paid for?
- What do you not enjoy about what you do that you don't get paid for?
- What do you do to rest and recuperate?
- What do you enjoy about what you do to rest and recuperate?
- What gets in the way of enjoying your rest and recuperation?
- In an average week, what percentage of your time do you devote to these three areas?

DEVELOPING FLOW

Csikszentmihalyi (2002, p 3) notes that '*the best moments usually occur when a person's body or mind is stretched to its limits in voluntary effort to accomplish something difficult and worthwhile*'. This requires a state of 'flow' where the person is engaged in the task to the exclusion of all other tasks so that nothing else seems to matter. If we accept that work–life balance as it is traditionally constructed isn't what we are trying to achieve, then Csikszentmihalyi suggests that in order to free ourselves from the psychological binds the idea creates we must find reward in each moment. If we gain pleasure and satisfaction from the ongoing stream of our lives, then '*the burden of social controls automatically falls from our shoulders*' (Csikszentmihalyi, 2002, p 19). We are living a rich life in every moment of it. This 'flow' comes from being absorbed in the moment whatever we are doing to the exclusion of other things that are trying to draw our attention. This relies on having a trusted system that contains everything that is in our sphere of responsibility so that we are not burdening ourselves worrying about 'next things' but rather we are engrossed in the current thing. The trusted system is something we can return to when we are finished with one moment to see what needs to be done in the next. I talk about this in Chapter 7.

SELF-DETERMINATION THEORY

Self-determination theory, developed by Deci and Ryan (Pink, 2009), suggests we have three innate psychological needs that drive our satisfaction in the things we do. They are competence (or mastery), autonomy and relatedness. They suggest that when we cannot satisfy these needs our productivity, motivation and therefore our happiness reduce. There is a direct link between being productive and our happiness. We delight in a job done that motivates us on to the next job. This is because our desire to be self-determining and autonomous is innate. Being in control motivates us. We need to create conditions where we are able to learn about what is around us and be in a position psychologically to engage with it. This will promote our competence. We need conditions where we are able to make decisions for ourselves. For social workers this maybe isn't about next steps with service users, as that may often need some form of authorisation, but rather it's about being autonomous in how we do what we do. It is about how we do the job to get to the point where someone has to agree a decision. That is the bit we can be autonomous in. I'd argue that social work is a job that has the potential to afford its workforce a great deal of autonomy if we would stop tying practitioners up in bureaucracy. Finally, the job is all about relatedness, or should be. How we relate to service users, our colleagues and other professionals is crucial to getting the job right. So social work has the potential to fit with our innate drives and promote a healthy, happy workforce. The question of why it often doesn't is cause for concern. That undoubtedly warrants further exploration and research. For us here, in this book, we are going to think about what helps us stay well and helps us focus on what there is to do, no matter what the circumstances.

RESILIENCE

Resilience is multi-faceted. The importance of emotional resilience cannot be overestimated (Grant and Kinman, 2014). But the importance of physical resilience also cannot be overestimated, given the apparent impact of exercise and nutrition on productivity. Social workers, in fact all professionals, also need resilient 'being organised' systems to ensure they are organisationally resilient on a practical level, especially given the information and knowledge work that social workers engage in. We need to take care of all three elements – our physical resilience, our practical resilience and our emotional resilience – in order to stay well and be productive.

Emotional resilience

The risk of not being able to manage your own emotions while you work professionally with the emotions of others is that this can be an antecedent to personal ill health, both physical and mental, as we shall see throughout the book. It also leads to compassion fatigue, an indifference to the suffering or problems of others. Being in an emotionally demanding job can lead to a stress response which in turn can lead to 'burnout', outlined by Kinman et al (2014) as emotional exhaustion, a cynical outlook and a decline in personal accomplishments. This has an inevitable impact on productivity and how you relate to your clients. Ingram (2015) points out that reflection and support are key to building emotional resilience. Such support could be through quality supervision that moves beyond 'what next' case discussion and explores practitioners' emotions as a response to what they have observed in practice. He also notes though that we shouldn't simply dwell on negative emotions but should also explore positive emotions as they celebrate the profession and fuel a sense of role and identity. Consideration of emotions helps people reconnect with intrinsic motivators that initially drove their desire to study social work and should continue to drive them in post-qualifying practice. Throughout the coming chapters we shall see how all manner of things impact on our emotional well-being.

Physical resilience

Cannon (2018) states that to promote greater capacity to cope with stress we need to include exercise and relaxation into weekly lifestyle routines. Exercise has positive stress-busting effects, as we shall see in Chapter 4, and relaxation allows for recuperation. Chatterjee (2018, p 152) observes that engaging in exercise should be straightforward, pointing out that *'the world is your gym'*. All too often, people are locked into a view of exercise that emerged with the keep-fit craze of the 1980s and that sits engagement in exercise outside of usual day-to-day life and as something set apart to be done in special clothes in special places. This immediately places obstacles in the way of people and leads to inaction. '*I need a gym membership*', '*I need to book a class*', '*I need the latest training shoes.*' This is not the case. Physical exercise needs to be a part of routine life. Simple changes have big effects. In Chapter 4, we'll talk about the significant benefits of a 20-minute lunchtime walk.

The other part of physical resilience is nutrition. From Hippocrates in ancient Greece, who reportedly felt food was medicine, to Gillian McKeith, nutritionist and TV show host in the 1990s, we have been told that we are what we eat! Increasingly this is being shown to be true, with very recent research supporting the idea that the gut biome – the bacteria in our gut – plays an important role in moderating mood. Enders (2015) even goes as far as to suggest that our construction of our idea of 'self' is determined by the brain drawing on information and feelings from every part of the body including the gut. This brings the impact of physical 'feelings' into the creation of self – you are what you feel as a consequence of what you eat. We will explore some of this in Chapter 3.

Practical resilience

We work in a complex environment full of information that needs to be controlled so that we know what to do with it. We inhabit a working world where the idea of ever being 'caught up' is probably unrealistic and which therefore demands we know what there is to do so that we can figure out what it is we should do next. We also need to control those uncompleted tasks. We need systems that support us in the 'doing' and 'remembering' as there's too much to handle in our brain alone. Allen (2015) says that we cannot 'plan' and 'do' at the same time. We need a space to take stock followed by a period of activity. Heylighen and Vidal (2007) note that by unburdening memory into a trusted system that prompts you to take action, anxiety, and therefore stress, can be reduced. Taking a consistent approach to figure out what there is to do and then to plan doing it can indeed create the sense of 'flow' that Csikszentmihalyi (2002) considers as being essential for control, focus and well-being. This is in contrast to the world that we can all inhabit at times of information overload that leads to confusion and anxiety that in turn leads to procrastination that in turn leads to more anxiety (Heylighen and Vidal, 2007). This is a self-fuelling loop that saps our psychological capacity to 'do'. We need a plan. A good day starts the previous day, a good week, the previous week, and a good month, the previous month. In Chapter 7 we'll explore this.

WHAT IS SELF-CARE?

It is not by chance that we find ourselves at this time in human history talking about and being interested in well-being. Advances in neuroscience, together with psychology's increasing interest in the positive aspects of mental health, rather than solely the negative, have led to increased research into the relationship between physical and mental health and well-being (Webb, 2017). The importance of maintaining practitioner well-being cannot be overestimated, as stress, as we have seen, can lead to a lack of interest or empathy with the service user's position – compassion fatigue, burnout, self-doubt and interpersonal conflict in the workplace (Adams et al, 2006; Graham and Shier, 2014). Social work regulators demand of their registrants an understanding of maintenance of health and well-being, the ability to manage the physical and emotional impact of practice and identify and apply strategies to build professional resilience. This surely has to be undertaken within a partnership between the employer and the employee?

There is an important relationship between environmental, organisational and individual factors when considering the well-being of social work practitioners and exploring how they self-care to enhance resilience (Antonopoulou et al, 2017). Resilience, well-being promoted through self-care, and the activities engaged in to promote these things are personally defined (Graham and Shier, 2014) and initiated but there also needs to be a person-centred approach to supporting people in the workplace. Organisational change may be required to create the appropriate environment. This has been demonstrated in companies which have a keen focus on productivity and includes such things as opportunities for exercise, meditation and even naps (Levitin, 2015). As in social work practice, the voice of the individual needs to be the starting point.

Self-care is '*the practice of activities that individuals initiate and perform on their own behalf to maintain life, health, and well-being*' (Grafton and Coyne, 2012, p 17). Such activities need to be driven by internal motivation. Self-care is firstly about attending to ourselves. By attending to ourselves we create inner order. Secondly, we need to attend to the things that are in our sphere of responsibility. These will be things that need planning and organising and then doing. By attending to these things, we create order in our sphere of responsibility. Finally, we can decide what we let into our sphere of responsibility from the chaos outside of it. Where we can't control some of the chaos infiltrating our order, we need to develop a mind like water (Allen, 2015). When a rock is thrown into a perfectly still pond it creates ripples. Eventually the pond 'controls' the ripples as the stone settles on the bottom of the pond and the pond becomes perfectly still again. This is what we are trying to achieve in our lives. When something is thrown at us, we take it and order it, returning to a calm state after a period of activity to get it under control. Jordan Peterson puts it more beautifully:

> When things break down, what has been ignored rushes in. When things are no longer specified, with precision, the walls crumble, and chaos makes its presence known. When we've been careless, and let things slide, what we have refused to attend to gathers itself up, adopts a serpentine form, and strikes – often at the worst possible moment.
>
> (Peterson, 2018, p 266)

Self-care is engaging in a combination of activities that promote our well-being, give us a sense of order and control and give us the psychological and physical capacity to respond positively to life. The chapters of this book will help us explore the important elements that define our self-care canon.

REFLECTIVE TASK

What do you do to self-care?

When you think about this question, think about the things that you use to self-care that might be positive (for example, going for a walk) and negative (for example, drinking alcohol). Make two columns.

Think about the positive and negative impact on your well-being of the things in both columns.

THE KEY ELEMENTS OF SELF-CARE

There are three key elements to self-care that influence our resilience and productivity. They are sleep, exercise and nutrition. All have a chapter in the book. Sleep is deliberately at the bottom of the triangle (see diagram on page 149) as it is the foundation that all self-care starts from. In order to engage in these self-care elements, we need to 'be organised'. This being organised stretches across our whole lives, including the things we get paid to do, the things we do but don't get paid for and our recuperation. We need to think of all of these elements holistically as they all impact on each other. When we are tired, we are less likely to be motivated to exercise. When we have an afternoon slump we reach for sugary snacks. When we eat badly, or late at night, we don't sleep well. If we aren't organised, we feel stressed and our body reacts by producing cortisol and adrenaline. If we don't exercise, we don't 'burn' these chemicals up that were produced to prepare us for 'fight or flight'. If we don't sleep well, we can't muster the energy to make plans and be organised. And on it goes in a co-dependent cycle. We need to break negative cycles and produce positive ones. We need to understand that what we eat, how we sleep, the exercise we take and being organised all have the potential to prepare us for productive lives lived to the full. Peterson puts it eloquently when he says *'the body, with its various parts, needs to function like a well-rehearsed orchestra. Every system must play its role properly,'and at exactly the right time, or noise and chaos ensue'* (Peterson, 2018, p 18).

Having 'agency' is having a sense that you are causing, through deliberate action, the things that go on around you. This gives you a sense of control. It is the opposite to feeling helpless. Even if you do feel helpless in some areas there are still things you can have agency over (Hanson, 2018). When your options are very limited, look for the little things you *can* do, and focus on the feeling of agency regarding them. Build on that. But start to build. I hope in this book we will give you actionable things so you feel you can have some agency over the work you do and the care you take of yourself. That's what we want to achieve. There is a 'healthy worker effect' whereby people who are more robust stay in stressful jobs for longer (Grant and Kinman, 2014, p 21). Social work, as a consequence of its person-facing nature, is stressful. You didn't study and qualify to be in this profession just to let the job take so much from you that you leave it. We want to help you create a robust and resilient 'you' so that you can enjoy the things you get paid to do, enjoy the things you do just because you love doing them, and delight in the things you do to rest and recharge.

REFERENCES

Adams, E R, Boscarino, J A and Figley, C R (2006) Compassion Fatigue and Psychological Distress among Social Workers: A Validation Study. *American Journal of Orthopsychiatry*, 76(1): 103–8.

Allen, D (2015) *Getting Things Done: The Art of Stress-free Productivity*. London: Piatkus.

Antonopoulou, P, Killian, M and Forrester, D (2017) Levels of Stress and Anxiety in Child and Family Social Work: Workers' Perceptions of Organizational Structure, Professional Support and Workplace Opportunities in Children's Services in the UK. *Children and Youth Services Review*, 76(May): 42–50.

Bent-Goodley, T B (2018) Being Intentional about Self-care for Social Workers. *Social Work*, 63(1): 5–6.

Cannon, E (2018) *Is Your Job Making You Ill?* London: Piatkus.

Chatterjee, R (2018) *The 4 Pillar Plan*. London: Penguin Random House.

Crawshaw, P (2012) Governing at a Distance: Social Marketing and the (Bio) Politics of Responsibility. *Social Science and Medicine*, 75(1): 200–7.

Csikszentmihalyi, M (2000) *Beyond Boredom and Anxiety*. San Francisco, CA: Wiley and Sons.

Csikszentmihalyi, M (2002) *Flow*. London: Rider (The Random House Group).

Davidson, L (2015) British Workers Are Skipping Lunch and That's Hurting Productivity. *The Telegraph*, 6 January 2015. [online] Available at: www.telegraph.co.uk/finance/jobs/11326076/British-workers-are-skipping-lunch-and-thats-hurting-productivity.html (accessed 4 February 2020).

Deacon, L (2017) Introduction. In Deacon, L and Macdonald, S J *Social Work Theory and Practice* (pp 1–10). London: Sage.

Enders, G (2015) *Gut: The Inside Story of Our Body's Most Underrated Organ*. London: Scribe.

Gibson, M (2017) Social Worker or Social Administrator? Findings from a Qualitative Case Study of a Child Protection Social Work Team. *Child and Family Social Work*, 22(3): 1187–96.

Grafton, C and Coyne, E (2012) Practical Self-care and Stress Management for Oncology Nurses. *The Australian Journal of Cancer Nursing*, 13: 17–20.

Graham, J R and Shier, M L (2014) Profession and Workplace Expectations of Social Workers: Implications for Social Worker Subjective Well-being. *Journal of Social Work Practice*, 28(1): 95–100.

Grant, L and Kinman, G (2014) What Is Resilience? In Grant, L and Kinman, G (eds) *Developing Resilience for Social Work Practice* (pp 16–30). London: Palgrave.

Grant, L, Kinman, G and Fountain, R (2014) Social Work and Wellbeing: Setting the Scene. In Grant, L and Kinman, G (eds) *Developing Resilience for Social Work Practice* (pp 3–15). London: Palgrave Macmillan.

Griffiths, M (2017) *The Challenge of Existential Social Work Practice*. London: Palgrave.

Guardian (2019) Heart Racing, Palms Sweaty – What Does Stress Do to the Body? [online] Available at: www.theguardian.com/lifeandstyle/2019/feb/04/stress-anxiety-knees-weak-palms-sweaty (accessed 4 February 2020).

Handy, C (1999) *Understanding Organizations* (4th ed). London: Penguin.

Hanson, R (2018) *Resilient*. London: Penguin Random House.

Health and Care Professions Council (2016) Gender Break Down of Social Workers in England – December 2016. [online] Available at: www.hcpc-uk.org/resources/freedom-of-information-requests/2017/gender-break-down-of-social-workers-in-england---december-2016/ (accessed 4 February 2020).

Healy, K (2014) *Social Work Theories in Context* (2nd ed). Basingstoke: Palgrave Macmillan.

Heylighen, F and Vidal, C (2007) Getting Things Done: The Science behind Stress-free Productivity. Brussels: Evolution, Complexity and Cognition Research Group (Free University of Brussels).

Heyns, T, Botma, Y and Van Rensburg, G (2017) A Creative Analysis of the Role of Practice Development Facilitators in a Critical Care Environment. *Health SA Gesondheid*, 22 (December): 105–11.

Hughes, M and Wearing, M (2017) *Organisations and Management in Social Work* (3rd ed). London: Sage.

Iacono, G (2017) A Call for Self-compassion in Social Work Education. *Journal of Teaching in Social Work*, 37(5): 454–76.

Ingram, R (2015) *Understanding Emotions in Social Work*. Maidenhead: Open University Press.

James, E, Mitchell, R and Morgan, H (2019) *Social Work, Cats and Rocket Science*. London: Jessica Kingsley.

Keller, G and Papasan, J (2014) *The One Thing*. London: John Murray.

Kinman, G, McDowell, A and Uys, M (2014) The Work/Home Interface – Building Effective Boundaries. In Grant, L and Kinman, G (eds) *Developing Resilience for Social Work Practice* (pp 33–53). London: Palgrave.

Levitin, D (2015) *The Organized Mind: Thinking Straight in the Age of Information Overload*. London: Penguin.

Luetchford, G (2015) 'If You Don't Take Care of Yourself, How Can You Possibly Help and Support Others?' [online] Available at: www.communitycare.co.uk/2015/05/13/dont-take-care-can-possibly-help-support-others/ (accessed 4 February 2020).

Marc, C and Osvat, C (2013) Stress and Burnout among Social Workers. *Social Work Review / Revista de Asistență Socială*, 12(3): 121–30.

Netting, F E, Kettner, P M and McMurty, S L (1993) *Social Work Macro Practice*. New York: Longman.

Peterson, J B (2018) *12 Rules for Life: An Antidote for Chaos*. Toronto: Random House.

Pink, D H (2009) *Drive: The Surprising Truth about What Motivates Us*. Edinburgh: Canongate.

Sánchez-Moreno, E, de La Fuente Roldán, I, Gallardo-Peralta, L P and López de Roda, A B (2015) Burnout, Informal Social Support and Psychological Distress among Social Workers. *British Journal of Social Work*, 45(8): 2368–86.

Skagen, K and Collins, A M (2016) The Consequences of Sickness Presenteeism on Health and Wellbeing over Time: A Systematic Review. *Social Science and Medicine*, 161 (July): 169–77.

Stacey, G, Aubeeluck, A, Cook, G and Dutta, S (2017) A Case Study Exploring the Experience of Resilience-based Clinical Supervision and Its Influence on Care towards Self and Others among Student Nurses. *International Practice Development Journal*, 7(2): 1–16.

Webb, C (2017) *How to Have a Good Day: The Essential Toolkit for a Productive Day at Work and Beyond*. London: Palgrave Macmillan.

Sleep: nutrition for the mind

Stephen

INTRODUCTION: WORK, PLAY, SLEEP, REPEAT

Of all the things in this book we are writing about, I have come to the conclusion there is one factor most instrumental in self-care, well-being and productivity – and that is sleep. I have heard the same phrase time and time again: '*If only I could get a good night's sleep, I feel I could face anything.*' I have heard this from practitioners, and I've heard it from family carers struggling to maintain their caring role. Sleep seems to be the cornerstone of any attempt to keep things together and on track. As we shall see, not only does a lack of sleep affect things like concentration, planning and analysing, it also has a profound physical effect on our bodies, making us more susceptible to ill health. Walker (2018) comments that for too long we have seen poor sleep as a symptom of conditions rather than the possible cause. We need to give that careful consideration.

Before the industrial revolution, workers were more attuned to night and day. We now understand how our bodies are locked into a circadian rhythm that relies on dark and light, as this helps the production of chemicals in our brains. The cues of it getting dark or light, along with other factors, initiate our sleep and waking. Picture our earlier lifestyles, living off the land, working while it was light, sleeping when it was dark. Without wanting to paint an idyllic picture of life in previous centuries, it is clear the trappings of modern life, and the opportunities that go with it, can get in the way of a good night's sleep.

The pattern culturally associated with how we sleep has changed since the advent of artificial light. We can now extend the daylight into the hours of dusk and brighten up early winter mornings at the flick of a switch. We used to have a bi-modal sleep pattern, sleeping for four or five hours early in the evening, usually after our last meal of the day, followed by one or two hours awake, and concluding with four or five hours of further sleep to get us to morning. This was also supplemented by an afternoon nap just like the siesta some cultures continue to enjoy today.

This pattern of sleep, particularly the afternoon nap, has been shown to be healthy for us, '*promoting greater life satisfaction, efficiency, and performance*' (Levitin, 2015, p 189). Companies at the cutting edge of this kind of knowledge, such as Nike and Google, provide nap rooms for employees. They know from NASA research that a 25-minute nap boosts performance by 34 per cent and alertness by 54 per cent (Webb, 2017). I suspect as busy practitioners you could do with that lift, but, equally, we are unlikely to see nap pods as a universal reality any time soon, which is a shame.

We have lost our bi-modal and afternoon nap pattern because we are locked into hours of working and ways of thinking about work and life outside of work. Using artificial light to extend our hours of activity means in some way we are working against our body's natural, instinctive way of functioning.

I am constantly amazed by the restorative nature of a good night of sleep. In so many circumstances I find myself thinking late on an evening, '*I can't do any more, I'm so tired I can barely move.*' I find myself physically exhausted. I could regale you with stories of epic bike rides or marathon runs that have left me physically with nothing left but I will save you that. Equally I can find myself psychologically or emotionally drained from the rigours of the working day and feel I just can't muster the energy to think about anything. But then, a good night's sleep, and we're fit to go again. Or at least should be.

THE LANGUAGE OF SLEEP

Sleep is embedded in our cultural psyche. When my wife and I wake up on a morning we invariably ask, '*How did you sleep?*' This is closely followed by '*Who is walking the dog?*' '*I slept like a baby*' is the response I love to hear to the '*How did you sleep?*' question. Because then I can say, '*What? You were up three times during the night crying and during two of them you had something to eat?*' and laugh at my own amazing sense of humour (because I'm a dad and that's what dads do).

'*I slept like a log*' is good response I often use myself. You didn't move, you fell asleep and didn't stir until the next morning. You were an inanimate object. This is interesting as it alludes to sleep being something in which there is nothing going on. As we shall find out, there is so much happening that is crucial to our well-being and that impacts on our productivity the next day. In some ways, being asleep is just as much an active time as being awake, except... you're asleep. Indeed, one well-used phrase we hear when we are pondering a difficult conundrum or big decision is 'sleep on it'. This seems to suggest something *is* going on while we are asleep as that decision somehow gets made, or that knotty issue resolved, while we are oblivious to the world around us.

The importance attributed to a good night's shuteye cannot be overestimated. You don't really need a chapter in a book to tell you how important it is because you know how you feel when you don't get a good night's sleep. Yet, lots of us often forgo what we know is good for us and that's a recurring theme every time we talk about any sort of self-care. So, keep reading... there's good stuff coming that will help you see the importance of this element of self-care and give you some ideas around promoting good sleep. We want to avoid the sluggish feeling that has you reaching for the coffee pot by mid-morning or sooner. We want to avoid you being no good to neither man nor beast by mid-afternoon.

Personally, for most of my life at least, I have been very lucky, and could 'fall asleep on a clothesline'. This fascinating phrase comes from the days of the workhouses of early twentieth century London where people who were homeless and couldn't afford the price of a bed for the night had made available to them a bench to sit on and a clothes line to lean over in order to sleep. Many people are less fortunate than me, however, and have problems with sleep. Matthew Walker (2018), drawing on his 20-year research career into sleep, suggests half of us are not getting as much sleep as we need. For most people who fall into the 'not sleeping well' category I'd imagine you are going to bed feeling tired and are unable to get to sleep because of what I refer to as the 'churn' of the day's activities. Or you may be thinking about tomorrow's tasks and have them going around and around in your head keeping you awake. 'Open loops', as David Allen (2015) refers to them. Things that you don't have recorded anywhere that you are trying to hang on to and remember. For me, having a 'trusted system' as outlined in the productivity chapter (Chapter 7) can help me to manage this to a large extent by knowing everything is captured, nothing is forgotten, and it's all just waiting there in an organised format, for me to get to it the next day. There are other people who fall asleep without problem but wake up in the early hours of the morning only to start to 'churn'. When I've got a lot going on this is what happens to me. I find some sort of mantra-like mindfulness exercise can help. I repeat *'there's nothing to be done now, this is my time'* over and over again until I drop off. It's a bit like counting sheep. (More on mindfulness in Chapter 5.)

Think about how you sleep

- What time do you usually go to bed?
- What time do you usually get up?
- Do you find it difficult to get to sleep?
- Do you wake up during the night?
- How do you feel when you wake up the next morning?
- Do you usually wake up naturally or does the alarm clock always wake you? Do you sleep differently on a weekend?

WHAT IS SLEEP?

In his lectures about dreams in 1915 Sigmund Freud asked the question *'What is sleep?'* and suggested that:

> *Sleep is a state in which I want to know nothing of the external world, in which I have taken my interest away from it. I put myself to sleep by withdrawing from the external world and keeping its stimuli away from me. I also go to sleep when I am fatigued by it. So when I go to sleep I say to the external world: 'Leave me in peace: I want to go to sleep.'*

(Freud, 1991 [1915], p 117)

Here Freud tells us, very simply, a few truths I feel are worthy of note. He talks about a state in which you have taken your interest away from the external world. I've already mentioned that what stops us getting to sleep is our attention on the external world, so we need to consider how we take our attention away from it in order to achieve rest. He also makes going to sleep a very personal responsibility. When I talk to people about self-care there is often a backlash, with people telling me, no matter what solutions I propose, that the problem is their workload or the nature of the work and is not about them wanting to disengage from it. I understand and accept this argument; however, I don't wholly agree with it. There are ways we can achieve distance, a 'settledness' about how we have left our work, in order to give us the space to engage in rest and recuperation, of which sleep is one part. Only the individual can take such actions. Many people work in stressful jobs and a proportion of them sleep well. So, while the job undoubtedly has an impact, and I am not denying workplace stress, I'm a great believer in doing something in the areas you can take responsibility for. My philosophy here is that I'm trying to be part of a solution rather than part of the problem. Only you can take action to work towards good sleep and good self-care, while you and others continue to make the case for organisational change around the other realities of professional practice.

Freud also talks about keeping the world's stimuli away. This proves so difficult with late night television, emails, smartphones and more. Part of having a good night's sleep is looking at how you prepare for sleep. There is compelling evidence that the light from our 'always-on' devices stimulates our brains and overturns the chemical process going on internally to facilitate sleep. The blue light (traditionally the sky when we were outdoors more) that sends an 'it's daytime' message to our brains is evident in such devices and has a negative impact on melatonin release essential for sleep. It has been discovered that melatonin release can be suppressed for 90 minutes after exposure to bright light (Webb, 2017). The number of people with sleep problems is increasing and for many it is the exposure to these bright artificial light sources that could be causing the problem. Exposure to a light level of 10,000 lux, which is approximately equal to being outside on a clear day, was shown to increase the length of time it took people to get to sleep in a Japanese study (Nakamura et al, 2019).

GETTING TO SLEEP

The desire to sleep is driven by the pineal gland's production of melatonin in your brain; the gland reacts to diminishing light by flooding your brain, making you feel sleepy and less alert. Melatonin starts to increase at around 9pm, then stays in your brain through the night for about 12 hours. It begins to fall to low levels when daylight seeps through your eyelids, 'instructing' the pineal gland to stop its production of melatonin, with levels being at their lowest around 9am. This cycle goes on in your body over a near to 24-hour cycle irrespective of what you are trying to push your body to do. In fact, this process is so chemically locked in that even in the absence of light the body continues this cycle.

Over 80 years ago in 1938, Professor Nathaniel Kleitman and his research assistant Bruce Richardson from the University of Chicago became their very own research project. They took a trip to Kentucky and entered Mammoth Cave with enough supplies to last them six weeks. Mammoth Cave is one of the deepest caves on the planet, so no light penetrates its depths. In the cave they set about living in darkness to see what happened. Their work established that we have a biological, circadian rhythm of about 24 hours, and it showed that in the absence of the external stimuli of light we do not descend into a chaotic random sequence of waking and sleeping. They discovered that they were awake for about 15 hours and then asleep for about nine hours. Does that sound familiar? They did, though, find that the human 'rhythm' is not precisely 24 hours. Later research building on their own showed that on average, if left alone, we work on a 'clock' of about 24 hours and 15 minutes. Thankfully, our in-built chemistry and our pineal gland keep us on track by utilising our reaction to light and dark and working alongside other factors such as a drop in core body temperature to get us to sleep. This gives us some clues to the ideal sleep pattern we are searching for.

QUANTITY AND QUALITY

The World Health Organization and the National Sleep Foundation tell us something I suspect you already know. We should be aiming for about eight hours of sleep per night. Certainly, we should be within the region of seven to nine hours. The World Health Organization has stated that sleep loss is now an epidemic in the industrial world and Walker (2018) states that:

> *Routinely sleeping less than six or seven hours a night demolishes your immune system, more than doubling your risk of cancer. Insufficient sleep is a key lifestyle factor determining whether or not you develop Alzheimer's disease. Inadequate sleep – even moderate reduction for just one week – disrupts blood sugar levels so profoundly that you would be classified as pre-diabetic…*
>
> (Walker, 2018, p 3)

A lack of sleep doesn't only affect your physical health; it also takes effect on your mental state. It can make you sluggish, prone to poor decision making and procrastination, and can impact on creative problem solving (Tuck, 2018). In professional practice clear decision making and effective problem solving are crucial to the role. Walker (2018) also suggests that lack of sleep doesn't necessarily throw us into a negative mood state but may well lead to a see-saw of emotions. He points out that any extremity of emotion, positive or negative, can be dangerous, stating that negative emotions can lead to feelings of worthlessness and a questioning of the value of one's life.

Surely, as professionals, we need to value ourselves first and value our contribution so that we can value the lives and contributions of others? While working with people often in a crisis themselves we need to be maintaining our own emotional stability, drawing on our emotional intelligence to facilitate a professional intervention. Howe (2008) notes that if our emotions are negative, we can become psychologically defensive, which can lead to us being absorbed in our own distress, potentially creating a lack of compassion.

It's not only the quantity of sleep we need to get right but also the quality of that sleep. During the night we go through different stages of sleep, all of which are essential. As we have seen above, our bodies are 'programmed' by the chemical reactions going on inside. If our brain chemistry is responding to the light–dark cycle, then we should sleep in tune with this cycle. As the level of melatonin is on the rise in our brains from about 9pm we should be trying to achieve a bedtime of between 10 and 10.30pm. Our eight hours of sleep would then take us to 6 to 6.30am, perfectly in sync with the rise and fall of melatonin governed by the available light. This needs to be developed as a routine night after night, seven days a week.

One of the things that always puzzles me is the way as parents we completely understand how giving babies and children routine is good for them. I remember as a parent, for my children, it was bath at 7pm, supper at 7.30, story at 7.45, bed at 8. And it works wonderfully for many. For some reason which we become adults, we laugh in the face of routine; yet intuitively I feel we know it works. This seems to be another one of those things we have knowledge of but do nothing with and then wonder why we are cranky in the morning.

Throughout the night we establish a pattern of two sorts of sleep – non-rapid eye movement (NREM) sleep and rapid eye movement (REM) sleep – which do different things. What is notable here is that throughout the night, in an approximately 90-minute cycle, we move between the two (there are actually four stages of NREM sleep but that's a little technical for what we need to know here). NREM sleep dominates the early part of the night and REM sleep dominates the later part of the night, or early morning, depending on how you want to look at it. These two forms of sleep are crucial to memory storage.

Walker (2018) describes the need for this pattern beautifully, using the metaphor of a sculptor working a block of clay. To start with, all of the raw material is available to him, the same way all of our memories from the day are stored in our short-term memory. The sculptor then starts by deciding what superfluous matter can be removed, what pieces of clay are not required. During this period, early details are made. Finer structures are then worked on to reveal details and 'store' those details in the beauty of the finished sculpture. If we apply this to sleep, the early part of sleep (NREM) helps us with the processing of information and making the big decisions about what is important. Unnecessary information is discarded with a little transfer of details. REM sleep, which comes later in the night, deals with the details and the storage of these memories. It is the REM sleep that does the work of forging connections with older memories and it is during this period we dream.

Your brain is trying to achieve this process whether you are awake or asleep based on the biological rhythms controlling your brain. Being awake gets in the way of this being successful. So, as we have seen, your brain is ready to start work on this at around 10pm and needs to be done by about 6am. If you decide to stay up until 2am to binge watch the latest TV series, you have lost that early NREM heavy/REM light sleep, meaning there's been no culling of the big information to leave you with the finer details. If you need to get up at 4am to get the train for a meeting at 9am then your brain hasn't finished achieving what it needs to do in the REM heavy/NREM light sleep period. Either of these scenarios is compromising your ability to store memories and make connections with older memories. This process, in Walker's words, is like pressing 'save' on your computer and is therefore crucial. This was shown to great effect in a study by Ji and Wilson (2007) from MIT's Picower Institute for Learning and Memory. He showed that rats presented with a maze that led to rewards repeated the same patterns of brain activity when asleep as they had when engaged in the task, encoding this important memory from the day so it could be recalled.

What this also shows is that sleeping less during the week and trying to catch up on a weekend doesn't work. Trying to buy back sleep by having a lie in on a weekend doesn't offset those lost hours. *'The brain can never recover all the sleep it has been deprived of'* (Walker, 2018, p 297).

PRODUCTIVITY IMPACT

Lack of sleep leads to lack of productivity, with typically lower work rates and therefore slower completion of tasks. It is estimated that lost productivity in America costs between $2,000 and $3,500 per sleep-deprived employee per year. This is as a consequence of being less happy and lacking in motivation. Sleep-deprived people can be volatile, rash and prone to making poorly conceived decisions, because lack of sleep impacts on the frontal lobe, the part of the brain that manages our emotional impulses and mediates our self-control. Broken or disturbed sleep is also problematic and can lead to lower activity in the prefrontal cortex of the brain according to Schilpzand et al (2018). The impact of this is poor cognitive processing, planning and problem solving. Moreover, Schilpzand et al (2018) discovered that sleep-deprived workers shy away from setting themselves proactive goals in terms of complex work, defaulting to easier options. The risk, I'd suggest, here is that difficult tasks are deprioritised repeatedly until finally they must be done. This is often last minute, at the end of the day when our brain resources are at their lowest and needing to be 'recharged' by sleep. Not the best way to be working on important tasks!

We can understand then how lack of sleep is a dangerous business… and dangerous for our business (Walker, 2018). Our 'business' is work with vulnerable people often in a state of heightened emotions themselves, needing us to be in charge of our own emotions to be effective practitioners.

Think about a time when you had not had much sleep

- How did it make you feel?
- What strategies did you use to get through the day (positive or negative)?
- How productive were you?

CHRONOTYPE

It's worth mentioning here that how we respond to the onslaught of the day is different for all of us, as we are all a particular chronotype. We respond to the relentless march of the clock differently. Some of us are morning larks and some of us are night owls. Thinking about what chronotype you are can have a dramatic effect on your productivity and how you work. I'm a morning person. I'm good from about 6am to about 11am when I tend to get a slump. Getting outside and having some lunch invigorates me then I'm good from about 1pm to 3pm. But after 3pm… don't ask me to do anything that requires me to think!

Some people are the opposite and take a lot of time to get going. Now, I can't simply leave work at 3pm, citing my chronotype as the protagonist in my early departure, but what I have done is constructed a way of working that plays to my strengths. I try, as far as I can, to do my writing and thinking work on a morning in the 6am to 11am window. Then, less challenging tasks that still require thought I do from 1pm to 3pm. When I hit 3pm then it's simply routine admin tasks like printing documents ready for tomorrow and the week ahead, straightforward phone calls and appointment making, photocopying, or data entry type tasks. I do a lot of planning in the later part of the day as this means I leave with everything in order ready for the next day. I'm not saying planning is easy but it's not as difficult as writing a report or reading complex information. More on productivity in Chapter 7.

CAFFEINE AND ALCOHOL

If the statistics are right, every second person reading this is sleep deprived to one extent or another. One remedy we tend to turn to is caffeine. Caffeine disrupts the ability of a chemical called adenosine to latch on to receptors in your brain. Adenosine's job is to create what is termed sleep pressure, a force determining how sleepy you feel. The caffeine stops this chemical effect by latching on to the receptors instead. The problem is the adenosine in your brain continues to accumulate just waiting for its chance to invade the receptors. Once your body has removed the caffeine, using enzymes in your liver, the adenosine rushes in and you get that almighty mid-afternoon coffee slump. So, to offset this, as you feel it taking place, you drink more coffee, or tea (normal or green), or caffeinated drinks, or eat chocolate – all of which usually include caffeine. This can have a knock-on effect later when you are trying to get to sleep. The half-life of caffeine (the amount of time it takes your body to deal with 50 per cent of the drug) is five to seven hours. So that cup of coffee you have at 6pm is only halfway out of your 'system' by midnight. And be warned, 'decaff' is not 'no caff'. There is still about 15 to 20 per cent of the amount of caffeine in there compared to a standard cup.

Alcohol is not helpful in promoting good quality sleep either and falling asleep after a few drinks is not giving us the quality of sleep we need. While many of us can report falling asleep easily after a few alcoholic drinks the reality is alcohol is a sedative. So, you are sedated rather than asleep, and this disrupts the NREM and REM pattern we've already explored. Alcohol makes sleep fragmented so it '*is therefore not continuous and, as a result, not restorative*' (Walker, 2018, p 271).

THE IMPACT OF GOOD SLEEP

Sleep helps to maintain both physiological and psychological function. Here again we see the link between the three elements of the self-care triangle. In order to exercise effectively we need to be maintaining adequate sleep. In order to maintain focus on sound nutritional intake we need to have the psychological energy to do so. In terms of the overarching concept of 'being organised' we need to be able to apply all of our psychological functioning to the mental effort of the day.

The result of a lack of both the right quantity and the right quality of sleep is poor attention, poor planning, diminished cognitive functioning and poor judgement. The impact on our productivity as a consequence of poor sleep cannot be overstated. Research has shown that just one night when you sleep for a maximum of four hours can make you so sleep deprived you are more likely to make errors and be less attentive (Nakamura et al, 2019). Now imagine the number of mistakes you'd make if you were having less than our eight hours of sleep night after night.

Many work-based cultures almost celebrate the sacrifice of sleep, applauding people who work late and turn in early. But a week of reduced sleep can create an impairment in functioning the equivalent of a 0.1 per cent blood alcohol level, similar to being drunk. You wouldn't put yourself behind the steering wheel of a car under those circumstances, yet are left to make important decisions, about other people's lives, while experiencing the same level of impairment as intoxication.

A bad night's sleep can also affect your IQ level by a few points. On the other hand, a good night's sleep has been shown in research at the University of California Berkeley to make people twice as effective at spotting complex patterns in information; the research has also shown that people are able to solve 30 per cent more anagrams after a period of rest that included REM sleep (Webb, 2017). Sleep improves our cognitive function and skills like analysis and critical thinking.

Barber et al (2014) found better sleep practices could reduce the negative feelings people experience when placed under stress. People may respond less negatively towards the circumstances of the day when well rested and respond better to the rigours of the job. Also, better sleep may actually increase how much people feel in control of the stressful situations they encounter. This is possibly as a consequence of how much energy they feel they have to confront the situation, be that either psychological or physical energy, or both.

Schulz and Burton (2018, p 1640) state that a study of nearly 600,000 adults in a range of industries showed '*Employees who achieved optimal sleep levels of 7 to 8 hours per night had the lowest average number of health risk factors, the smallest productivity losses, and lower odds of having several health conditions compared to poor sleepers.*' Surely then there is a role for us on an individual level to take care of ourselves but also for employers to invest in education for their staff about sleep. Businesses and organisations need to take a careful look to see if the working environment they have established is impacting negatively on the sleep of their staff and consider changes to ensure it is supportive of good sleep practices. While I believe self-responsibility is so important to self-care, organisations need to accept the impact of professional roles and also support staff in appropriate ways.

If we can achieve good sleep what can we expect? Dr Rangan Chatterjee, in his '4 Pillar Plan' (2018), gives us the following list of benefits of a good night's sleep:

- increased energy;
- improved concentration;
- greater capacity to learn;
- better ability to make healthy food choices;
- improved immune system function;
- enhanced autophagy (the way the body clears out damaged cells);
- better memory;
- increased life expectancy;
- reduced risk of being overweight;
- reduced stress levels;
- reduced risk of developing chronic disease eg type 2 diabetes and Alzheimer's.

(Chatterjee, 2018, pp 206–7)

SOUND ADVICE

The National Health Service (NHS, 2016) offers some simple, straightforward advice to improve your sleep environment and practices that may help. It would be useful to look at each of the ideas in turn.

Keep to a regular bedtime routine

Remember it's not just babies that need a routine, it's any human being. Much as we kick against it as adults, we are creatures of habit and routine. Your body is programmed into a chemical routine that does its best to achieve sleep, rest and waking. And what do we do? We ignore it! We stop up late and wonder why we are tired the next day. We get up late and wonder why we then can't get to sleep the next night. We self-medicate with alcohol and caffeine to get that little bit more out of the day and out of our social life. Someone once said to me, '*Drinking coffee steals hours from later in the day and drinking alcohol steals hours from tomorrow!*' All we achieve is the disruption of our programmed chemical clock and when we don't attend to it for long enough the situation becomes chronic. You should establish a pattern of sleep that fits your biological clock and you should maintain it seven days a week, 365 days a year.

Sleep at regular times

This will train your brain and internal body clock, aligning you to a natural sleep pattern. As we've seen, we need around eight hours of sleep a night and we should be sleeping from about 10pm to 10.30pm until 6am to 6.30am. These timings are in tune with our natural rhythm. So that's your starting point.

Don't go to bed hyped

While exercise is an important aspect of self-care (see Chapter 4) you should avoid it for two or three hours before bedtime. A good way to wind down is to have a warm bath – again, isn't that part of the routine we give babies? There's a drop in your core body temperature orchestrated by your circadian rhythm's signal 'time to sleep', and it reaches its low point about two hours after sleep onset, which remember starts at about 9pm. This drop in temperature happens whether you actually achieve sleep or not, which is why people often feel cold when tired. Having a hot bath seems counter-intuitive and seems to be going against this tide your body is creating. But it's not. The hot bath draws blood to the surface of your body and when you get out of the bath the dilated blood vessels on the surface disperse heat causing your core temperature to drop, which leads to feeling sleepy.

Write 'to do' lists for tomorrow

One of the main things that keeps people awake is trying to remember things they need to do tomorrow. Before you go to bed (or ideally at the end of your working day – see

Chapter 7 on productivity), write down everything you need to do the next day, safely leaving your notes in a place you can find them when you need to, without having them going round and round in your head. Keep a notepad by your bed. If you think of something while in bed, write it down. There's good evidence externalising memories in this way can help us 'put them to bed' to help put us to bed.

Do relaxation exercises such as yoga or listen to relaxation CDs

There is a huge range of yoga and relaxation CDs and apps available that might help you. Anything that calms your mind and distracts you from your racing thoughts. You could try audio books, or read a book, or maybe listen to the radio. You should avoid TV and smartphones as not only do they stimulate your brain, but the light they emit confuses your brain into thinking it is daylight. One way to improve sleep quality could be through mindfulness practice (see Chapter 5). Results from a study by Hulsheger et al (2015) showed that some brief self-training in mindfulness practice not only increased mindfulness during work but also improved sleep quality and sleep duration.

Your bedroom should be a relaxing environment

It may sound obvious, but have the best mattress and pillows you can afford. Try different numbers of pillows and different types. You may find a harder or softer pillow helps. You should keep your bedroom for sleep (and sex... unlike most other vigorous activity, sex makes you sleepy!). Avoid distractions like TVs and ticking clocks. Buy an old-fashioned alarm clock and leave your smartphone somewhere else. Keep the room tidy, make your bed when you first get up, so, when you eventually get to bed after a hard day, it looks clean and inviting. Your bedroom should be cool (between 18 and 24 degrees centigrade – but go low) and dark. There should be no glowing lights from inside or outside the bedroom.

We can all benefit from improving the quality of our sleep. For many of us, it may simply be a case of making small lifestyle or attitude adjustments in order to help us sleep better (O'Sullivan, 2016). While these ideas are effective for many, you do need to give them a good month or so to see improvements.

Some people, no matter what they do, find sleeping problems continue, so I would advise you to seek medical advice. But do be mindful of the concern raised by Walker (2018) about prescription drug-induced sleep which, in his view, aids sedation rather than instigates good quality sleep. This means you feel you have been asleep but have missed many of the benefits. Your GP should be able to refer you to sleep specialists rather than simply prescribing or recommending medication. On a final note, you may find it useful to keep a sleep diary while making changes. This should detail what you have done during the day, how you have prepared for sleep, what time you went to bed, what it is that is keeping you awake and how often you do wake, what time you get up and how you feel when you do. Make sure you document as much as you can as your GP will need this information if you do seek medical advice.

REFERENCES

Allen, D (2015) *Getting Things Done: The Art of Stress-free Productivity*. London: Piatkus.

Barber, L K, Rupprecht, E A and Munz, D C (2014) Sleep Habits May Undermine Well-being through the Stressor Appraisal Process. *Journal of Happiness Studies*, 15: 285–99. Published online, 26 February 2013. doi:10.1007/s10902-013-9422-2.

Chatterjee, R (2018) *The 4 Pillar Plan*. London: Penguin Random House.

Freud, S (1991) [1915] *Introductory Lectures on Psychoanalysis*. London: Penguin.

Howe, D (2008) *The Emotionally Intelligent Social Worker*. Basingstoke: Palgrave Macmillan.

Hulsheger, I R, Feinholdt, A and Nubold, A (2015) A Low-dose Mindfulness Intervention and Recovery from Work: Effects on Psychological Detachment, Sleep Quality, and Sleep Duration. *Journal of Occupational and Organizational Psychology*, 88(3): 464–80. doi:10.121211/joop.12115.

Ji, D and Wilson, M A (2007) Coordinated memory replay in the visual cortex and hippocampus during sleep. *Nature Neuroscience*, 10(1): 100–7.

Levitin, D (2015) *The Organized Mind: Thinking Straight in the Age of Information Overload*. London: Penguin.

Nakamura, Y, Choi, Y, Akazawa, N, Park, I, Kawana, F, Satoh, M, Tokuyama, K and Maeda, S (2019) The Effect of Sleep Quality on Cognitive Functions in Young Healthy Men. *Advances in Exercise and Sports Physiology*, 24(4): 51–5.

NHS (National Health Service) (2016) How to Get to Sleep. [online] Available at: www.nhs.uk/live-well/sleep-and-tiredness/how-to-get-to-sleep/ (accessed 4 February 2020).

O'Sullivan, C (2016) The Importance of Sleep. [online] Available at: www.mentalhealth.org.uk/blog/importance-sleep (accessed 4 February 2020).

Schilpzand, P, Houston, L and Cho, J (2018) Not Too Tired to Be Proactive: Daily Empowering Leadership Spurs Next-morning Employee Proactivity as Moderated by Nightly Sleep Quality. *Academy of Management Journal*, 61(6): 2367–87. [online] Available at: https://doi.org/10.5465/amj.2016.0936 (accessed 4 February 2020).

Schultz, A B and Burton, W N (2018) Sleep: An Integral Component of Employee Well-being Programs. *American Journal of Health Promotion*, 32(7): 1639–41.

Tuck (2018) Productivity and Sleep. [online] Available at: www.tuck.com/productivity-and-sleep/ (accessed 4 February 2020).

Walker, M (2018) *Why We Sleep*. London: Penguin Random House.

Webb, C (2017) *How to Have a Good Day: The Essential Toolkit for a Productive Day at Work and Beyond*. London: Pan Macmillan.

3 Nutrition: the impact of what you eat and drink

Lisa

INTRODUCTION: RUBBISH IN, RUBBISH OUT

One of the things I know and acknowledge about myself is I use food as a means of managing my emotions. Whatever is going on in my life, food is usually taking centre stage in some shape or form. When happy, I celebrate life's achievements and the fact life is good with food. This is usually in the form of cake or a meal out with loved ones so they can join me in my haze of happiness. I believe this stems from childhood, as my mother would reward good behaviour with sweet treats. On a spiritual level, I am also celebrating the sweetness of life.

When life is crashing and burning all around me, I commiserate with food. I wallow in self-pity and I know only too well it's the salty savouriness of crisps, or pizza takeaways, that will bring me the emotional comfort I crave at that time. Perhaps on a subconscious and spiritual level I am looking to make life more savoury and flavoursome when hitting that low point.

When I reflect upon how this pattern of behaviour impacts upon my time, energy and ability to think clearly at those critical moments, with a degree of level headedness, I understand how using food to regulate my emotions can be counterproductive.

Like Stephen, as he describes himself in his sleep chapter, I identify as being more productive on a morning. Mid-morning and afternoon energy slumps lead to a caffeine pick me up and a sugar rush from the biscuits and sweets lurking in the office. Go on, one won't hurt!

Once the immediate hit of artificial energy wears off, instead of being mentally alert and on the top of my game, I usually end up having an internal dialogue with my inner child. Digging my trouser waistband from my muffin top as I chastise her for yet again having so little will power when it comes to resisting all the yummy temptations lying around the office. Even our analogies are food based – 'muffin top'!

I'm sure you don't need reminding that our lives are more stressful now than ever before. If they weren't, we wouldn't have a theme for our book! We talk throughout the book about how many different things can impact upon our mental, emotional and physical health. In reality, can our nutritional habits really add to our stress? Unfortunately, yes.

EATING HEALTHILY

Here in the UK, it's not just me who loves food; 'we' are a nation of foodies, we simply love our food and drink. As Oscar Wilde reportedly said, '*After a good dinner, one can forgive anybody, even one's own relatives.*'

There is a significant body of research that shows that endless mugs of steaming coffee, processed meals and 'grab 'n' go' sandwiches, coupled with excessive drinking and eating, can end up creating preventable health conditions, such as obesity, heart problems, diabetes and reduced mental well-being (Fenton, 2017). With a little forethought, planning and being organised, we can actually use nutrition to promote our physical and mental well-being as well as help us manage our stress levels (mentalhealth.org.uk, 2017).

Personally, I view nutrition a bit like running a car. If we don't use the correct fuel, then how can we expect the car to run smoothly? No matter how we look at things, we simply cannot get away from the fact that our bodies need good nutrition.

HEALTHY GUT AND THE VAGUS NERVE

I once had a manager ask me what made me so sure an adult son was financially abusing his father. I told her I just had this 'feeling' in my gut, though I couldn't pinpoint anything at that time. I was later proved right and the case went to court. Our emotions are known to stem from the brain. If our gut feelings are in the stomach, is there a direct link between the brain and the gut? Yes. Have you ever heard of the vagus nerve?

The brain uses information from the gut sent through the vagus nerve to figure out how things are going. Giulia Enders (2015) likens it to reception at the company office receiving calls from workers in the field updating on their status. If things aren't going well in the field, it has an impact at head office. So, if things aren't good in the gut, then that has an impact on our emotions and therefore how we feel. Research shows that your gut biome (the bacteria in your intestines) is instrumental in gut health and has an impact on your mood and mental health to such an extent that some refer to your guts as the 'second brain'.

> *Always trust your gut.*
> *Your brain can be fooled.*
> *Your heart is an idiot.*
> *But your gut doesn't know how to lie.*
>
> (Author unknown)

Anderson and Yeo (2019) have explored how our gut biome 'health' affects our emotions. This is important as our emotions affect how we think and therefore how we feel psychologically. Enders (2015) also points out that about 80 per cent of our immune system is located in the gut. How diverse the microbes are in our gut directly affects our mood and our ability to fight disease. These things will obviously affect our productivity, and Cryan and Dinan (2012) report growing evidence that your microbiome influences your susceptibility to anxiety and depression.

Cryan (2019) repeated a Japanese experiment on sterile mice. These are mice bred with no microbiome (yes! Such things exist in the laboratory!). He showed, as the previous researchers had, that the gut biome had the 'power' to affect mood. In the initial sterile state, the mice showed symptoms of low mood and a stress response. They colonised the mice with 'good' gut bacteria and found their mood improved and their stress response diminished, evidence that the microbiome relieved stress.

An unhealthy diet can reduce these important signals and reduce the sensation of feeling full, which can lead to overeating. There are times when, even though my brain is busy, my stomach is crying out for food, so when that deadline looms it's so easy to grab whatever is in easy reach, especially in my office where sweets, chocolate and 'cake bake offs' are always on the go.

The vagus nerve

- The word 'vagus' means 'wandering' in Latin.
- It is one of the longest and most important cranial nerves in the body, running all the way from the brain stem to the colon.
- It is responsible for the regulation of internal organs, including those that regulate our digestion. So it helps the body get rid of food waste and absorb vital nutrients from the food we eat.

(Emeran et al, 2015)

Vagus nerve–brain relationship

This helps to:

- signal organs to create an inner-calm;
- 'rest-and-digest' during times of safety;
- prepare your body for 'fight or flight' in dangerous situations.

(Klarer et al, 2014)

Our gut biome is developed from the food broken down in our stomach as it passes through the gut. The nutrients from the food pass through small gaps in our intestinal wall and enter the bloodstream where they are transported to the various organs in the body. Each organ has its own function in terms of energy production, balancing hormones, promoting good skin integrity, positive mental well-being and the elimination of toxins and waste.

Within the gut there are hundreds of types of bacteria, some of which can be toxic. If the gaps in the gut wall become too wide, this can allow harmful bacteria to enter the blood stream. This is referred to as 'leaky gut' and has been identified as the main culprit in causing inflammation and as even being associated with depression (Kelly et al, 2015; Rooks and Garrett, 2016).

It is still not fully understood how leaky gut occurs, but a build-up of unhealthy bacteria produces excess gases and various other chemicals, resulting in bloating and stomach cramps. These gut bacteria thrive on foods such as sugar, dairy, gluten, soy and chemical additives found in processed foods, which in turn can affect your sleep and cause increased stress and anxiety.

It is claimed there are up to 1,000 species of bacteria in the human gut. Healthy bacteria such as *Lactobacillus* and *Bifidobacterium* (probiotics) can aid the digestion of certain food. They support the body to make the chemicals it needs to function at its optimum, working alongside the immune system and helping heal the gut (Lamprecht et al, 2012; Sender et al, 2016).

Leaky gut can cause:

- food intolerances;
- chemical sensitivity;
- excess gas;
- bloating, cramps;
- joint pain, headaches, brain fog, memory loss, fatigue, low mood and anxiety;
- reduction of the gut's ability to absorb vital nutrients;
- deficiencies in vital nutrients;
- energy decreases;
- inflammation;
- increased circulation of toxins;
- increased stress on the liver.

(NHS, 2018a)

PREBIOTICS AND PROBIOTICS

There is some evidence to suggest healthy gut bacteria such as *Lactobacillus acidophilusis*, one of the main probiotics, can help reduce cholesterol levels, as well as reduce abdominal pain associated with irritable bowel syndrome and boost the immune system (Cho and Kim, 2015; Kang et al, 2013; Sinn et al, 2008). *Bifidobacteria*, on the other hand, are believed to produce chemicals that can block harmful toxins from passing into the blood stream (Fukuda et al, 2011). In addition, they can also produce the chemical compounds controlling hunger, so are known to assist with weight loss (Ríos-Covián et al, 2016).

Studies have shown how probiotics can help stimulate vagus nerve activity, potentially leading to improved emotional well-being, especially in individuals with anxiety or depression (Hemarajata and Versalovic, 2013). Evidence from animal studies suggests healthy gut bacteria can increase the efficiency of communication between the brain and the vagus nerve, thus reducing stress-induced corticosterone levels present in anxiety-like and depression-like behaviour (Bravo et al, 2011).

Where can we find these good probiotics naturally?

We can find them in:

- fermented foods: sauerkraut, miso, tempeh, cheese, yoghurt;
- other foods: apples, almonds, bananas, barley, blueberries, cocoa, garlic, green tea, oats, onions, pistachios.

Apart from eating healthily we can support our healthy bacteria with prebiotics. Prebiotics are fibres found in food, fibres the body is unable to digest or absorb into the blood stream. In its simplest terms, these fibres are a valuable food source for healthy bacteria in the gut, combating inflammatory effects inside the colon. They also provide fuel to healthy cells so that they can grow and divide normally, thus reducing risk of developing cancerous cells (Segain et al, 2000).

Where can we find prebiotics naturally?

We can find them in:

- asparagus;
- bananas, berries;
- garlic, leeks;
- legumes, ie beans and peas;
- onions.

EMOTIONS AND EATING

I know what I eat and drink influences how I feel. When I overindulge on sugar, I have a stomping head all day. This means I struggle to concentrate at work and thus my productivity is reduced all day. Not good when you are trying to meet that deadline for a court report. Although the scientific relationship between food, the gut and mental well-being is in its infancy, we generally recognise intuitively that what we eat and drink can influence how we feel, think and behave (Cornah, 2006; McDonald, 2017). Growing evidence shows a direct link from our food and drink choices to an impact on what we think, how we feel, and therefore how productive we are at home and at work.

The mid-morning and mid-afternoon 'spike and crash' cycle of coffee and sugar might temporarily defeat the energy slump but does little to provide the correct fuel our body needs to function at its optimum. Remember the car I referred to earlier? Have you ever put diesel in a petrol tank? If you have, then you learned the hard way that you've got to get your fuel right or you damage your engine. Not taking on board the best fuel for your body will make it, and your brain, cough and splutter.

Poor nutrition can lead to reduced mental well-being according to The Royal College of Psychiatrists (RCP, 2015). It is useful to understand that stress influences our emotions, which in turn influences our thinking, which then influences our behaviour.

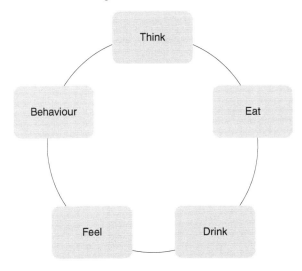

When I'm in a good mood (feel) I eat to celebrate (behaviour). This makes me feel good. But then I start to feel disappointed in myself (think) because of that fact I've just eaten unhealthily. This makes me feel low (feel) and to help make myself feel better I eat (behaviour). There are other examples. For some, drinking alcohol (drink) leads to snacking (eat) which leads to how you think and feel which influences your behaviour. You will certainly have your own experiences of these links I'm sure.

Stress is usually the underlying factor that leads us to reach for high-calorie foods. This is because when feeling stressed or anxious our bodies release high levels of cortisol. As we've discussed in other chapters, cortisol is a 'stress hormone' that leads to our primitive 'fight or flight' response in the face of danger. Specifically, in relation to nutrition it increases insulin levels in the body leading to a drop in blood sugar, which is why you end up craving sugary, high-fat foods. This is the body's way of getting you to eat high-calorie food to increase the body's fuel reserves in order to manage the impending surge of energy it is expecting in terms of needing to run from a dangerous situation (flight) or stand and face the danger head on (fight).

Just because our conscious selves know the danger is not necessarily a sabre-toothed tiger blocking the exit of our cave but rather a report that needs writing or a phone call that needs to be made, our primitive automatic response does not differentiate. Stress is stress. The downside of this efficient response from this machine we call the 'body' is that cortisol also increases the likelihood of the body storing fat, just in case we do have future encounters with sabre-toothed tigers!

More stress → more cortisol → increased appetite for junk food → more belly fat
(Talbott, 2007)

So, while we are biologically driven to food or drink as a means of coping with our stress, the impact can be potential weight gain which may leave you feeling worse. Then, when you feel negative about yourself you eat. This makes you feel low, so you eat to make yourself feel better. It's a vicious cycle: weight gain, reduced mental alertness, feeling low, reduced productivity, eat to feel better, and so the cycle continues. After a time, I get fed up with myself, I become focused and determined to kick my poor food habits once and for all. I decide I am going 'to be good' and explore how I can make long-term food changes as means of promoting my overall longevity, health and well-being. Tom Waterfall (2018) hits the nail on the head when he argues that, when making healthy eating changes, people tend to focus upon the long-term health benefits. It doesn't really cross our minds that small, simple changes can actually have quick results in terms of productivity.

Did you know that unhealthy eating has been linked to a 66 per cent increased risk of loss of productivity? Employees who rarely eat fruits, vegetables and other low-fat foods at work are 93 per cent more likely to have a higher loss in productivity (Merrill, 2012). The *British Journal of Health Psychology*, according to Ron Friedman (2014), found in one work-based study that increased consumption of fruits and vegetables by staff over a 13-day period actually resulted in them reporting feeling happier, more engaged and more creative than usual. It is likely that the increased intake of fruit and vegetables led to increased amounts of dopamine in the body, which is a neurotransmitter that enhances motivation and engagement. What does motivation and engagement result in? Increased productivity! Fruit and vegetables also contain antioxidants, known to improve memory and enhance mood, which means more motivation and engagement. What does motivation and engagement result in? Increased productivity! Get the picture? Next time work has you tearing your hair out, reach for the berries instead of the Terry's.

WHY IS GOOD NUTRITION IMPORTANT TO OUR BODIES?

It is clear good nutrition contributes to more than just good gut health. As Peterson (2018) says, the body is like an orchestra. Every part has its role to play to make beautiful music. If some parts aren't functioning well, then the music is discordant. It's the same with my previous car analogy. If not all the parts are working, then the car doesn't work well, or at all. Our bodies need a range of things to function well. Yurcheshen et al (2015) tell us we risk poor sleep–wake cycles, low mood and poor gut health if we are not eating the right things. This can lead to reduced productivity through fatigue, depression, anxiety and reduced sex drive.

Protein

The British Nutrition Foundation (BNF, 2018) explains how cells and tissues in the human body contain protein. Protein is needed as it enables growth, repair and general maintenance of our cells, tissue, cartilage and skin.

Protein deficiency leads to	Source
Muscle wastage, cramps, reduced wound healing, increased risk of infections. HumanN (2019)	Animal sources such as meat, fish, eggs and dairy products. Vegans and vegetarians can combine plant sources, ie pulses and cereals.

Carbohydrates

Carbohydrates, otherwise known as starch and sugar, are the main source of energy for the body (NHS, 2018b). Starch is needed in order to help produce the energy the body needs to function. I view starch as being fuel for the body in the same way petrol or diesel is to a car.

Sugar is also an important source of energy for our internal organs to function.

	Excess/deficiency	Source
Starch	Not enough intake of starch can lead to exhaustion, headaches, nausea, muscle cramps and reduced concentration.	Most foods contain some carbohydrates, but foods heavy in carbs tend to be potatoes, pasta, rice, lentils and wholemeal bread, as well as some fruits such as bananas.
Sugar	Sugar gives us that immediate mental boost, but can lead to a drop in glucose levels approximately 20 minutes later, which is why we can then become unfocused and easily distracted.	Sugar is found in fizzy drinks, breakfast cereals, biscuits, cakes, sweets, in fruits such as bananas, grapes and dates, and in honey.

Fat

You will no doubt be aware of how fat has had negative press for being bad for our over-all health. Yet we need fat in our diet as, like carbohydrates, fat is a source of energy (fuel) for our bodies. Fat helps maintain our core body temperature as well as aiding the absorption of some nutrients from our food (NHS, 2017a).

Saturated fat is the unhealthy fat, found in red meat, butter and other dairy products. Heart UK explain that saturated fats may raise cholesterol levels, which can lead to a build-up in the large blood vessels needed to carry blood around the body, thus increasing risks of developing coronary heart disease, angina and stroke (Heart UK, nd).

Monounsaturated and polyunsaturated are the two types of fat which are healthy for us.

	Excess	Source
Monounsaturated fats	Risk of high cholesterol levels leading to risk of coronary heart disease, angina and stroke.	Found in food sources such as avocados, almonds, cashews, peanuts and cooking oils made from plants or seeds (eg olives, peanuts, soybeans, rice bran, sesame and sunflower oils).
Polyunsaturated fats	Polyunsaturated fats include the type of fat known as Omega-3, deficiency of which can age the brain as well as reduce cognitive functioning. Omega-6 is another polyunsaturated fat, and without this we have increased risk of infections, excessive bleeding and poor skin regeneration.	Omega-3 is usually found in oily fish such as tuna, salmon and mackerel, while Omega-6 can be found in almonds, cashews, hazelnuts, peanuts, pecans, pistachios, eggs, edible seeds and corn or sunflower oil.

VITAMINS

Our bodies need a wide range of nutrients called 'vitamins' in order to maintain essential body processes such as healing wounds, boosting the immune system, giving us energy (always welcome when needing to get a job done in a tight timescale!) and repairing cellular damage. Without vitamins, we can end up exhibiting confusion, reduced concentration and lack of mental focus, among other health issues (NHS, 2017b).

Some vitamins are only soluble in fat and others in water. The body only needs a small number of vitamins, so I suppose you could liken this to the lubricants a vehicle needs to keep it ticking over, like water for the wipers, or engine oil, for example.

Fat-soluble vitamins

There are four fat-soluble vitamins, A, D, E and K, which are stored in the liver and fatty tissues. Their purpose is to aid healthy skin, bone repair, blood clotting and a healthy immune system (NHS, 2017b).

	Deficiency	Source
Fat-soluble vitamins	Increased risk of liver disease, excessive bleeding to wounds, brittle bones and weakened immune system leading to increased risk of opportunistic infections.	Vitamin D is the only vitamin the body makes for itself when the skin is exposed to sunlight. The others are found in animal products such as cheese, cream, butter, eggs, liver and oily fish, as well as leafy green vegetables (kale, spinach) and green vegetables (broccoli, brussels sprouts and asparagus).

Water-soluble vitamins

Water-soluble vitamins are not stored in the body and can only be consumed via our diet. The main water-soluble vitamins are B1, B2, B5, B6, B7 and B12, their purpose being to aid the body to change carbohydrates into energy. They also aid the body's ability to carry oxygen around the body as well as maintain good skin and hair.

Vitamins B9, V12 and V3 are also important for brain function, digestion and the nervous system. Vitamin C is important for wound healing, a healthy immune system and the maintenance of cartilage, bones and teeth (NHS, 2017b).

	Deficiency	Source
Water-soluble vitamins	Can lead to increased confusion, short-term memory loss, fatigue, depression, weakened immune system, respiratory infections, anaemia and skin problems.	Found in food sources such as: seafood, lean meat, poultry, dairy products, green vegetables (such as broccoli, brussels sprouts, spinach and asparagus), lentils, beans, nuts, seeds and sweet potatoes.

MINERALS

'*Eat your carrots or else you will never see in the dark*' is what I was always told by my mother as a child. Mind you, I won't go into details of the bribery required for me to eat sprouts! While I have little doubt most people will have heard of vitamins, I wonder whether the importance of minerals is as well known. We need minerals to help our body's overall function, including mental focus, alertness and prevention of fatigue (NHS, 2017b).

Minerals can be divided into two groups, major minerals and trace minerals. The major minerals are the ones our body needs more of, while for trace minerals we only need, well, a trace!

Major minerals

There are six major minerals, which are: calcium, chloride, potassium, sodium, magnesium and phosphorus.

As with vitamins, we need these major minerals for our bodies to function as the lean, mean racing machines we want them to be. Calcium, we know, is for healthy bone formation, but did you know it also helps with maintaining a regular heartbeat along with blood clotting?

Sodium, potassium and chloride also aid with balancing body fluids, including blood, in and around the cells, so they are important for stable blood pressure and protecting against strokes. Likewise, magnesium and phosphorus help the body to turn sugar and starch into energy as well as aiding good bone growth (NHS, 2017b).

	Deficiency	Source
Major minerals	The common results of deficiency for all the major minerals include: risk of osteoporosis (brittle bones), anxiety, fatigue, weakness, abnormal heart rhythm, high blood pressure, risk of strokes, lethargy and confusion.	All of these minerals can be found in table salt, olives and dairy products, such as milk and cheese. They can also be found in most vegetables, potatoes, sweet potatoes, nuts (ie peanuts, brazil, almonds), fish such as anchovies, sardines and salmon, shell fish such as prawns, and fruit such as tomatoes (yes, it's a fruit!), bananas and apples.

Trace minerals

While we may not require the likes of iron, zinc, iodine, fluoride, selenium and copper in as large amounts as our major minerals, our bodies do still need them to function well.

Iron and copper help the body form red blood cells and aid oxygen transportation to all major organs, as well as having a role in a healthy immune system and the production of essential hormones (such as cortisone and adrenaline!).

Zinc, selenium and copper help promote a healthy immune system and aid iron absorption, while iodine aids thyroid hormones and fluoride helps prevent tooth decay (NHS, 2017b).

	Deficiency	Source
Trace minerals	Common signs of deficiency can include: fatigue, weakness, reduced concentration, trouble learning or remembering and slower cognitive functioning, headaches, shortness of breath, heart palpitations, risk of brittle bones, clogged arteries, heart disease and strokes.	Most commonly found in meat, poultry, seafood, beans, nuts, brown rice, whole grains, vegetables, fruit, dairy products and dark chocolate.

There is so much information on the internet these days about nutritional requirements. I found the NHS website really useful and also came across the 'Eat Balanced' website, with interesting blogs, if you would like to check this out for yourself at: www.eatbalanced. com/why-eat-balanced/.

FOCUS, CONCENTRATION AND INCREASED PRODUCTIVITY

Did you know that while the brain is 2 per cent of an adult's weight, it actually uses 20 per cent of the body's energy? Tony Robbins (2019), an American motivational guru, explains how we can damage our brain cells through failure to follow a nutritious diet. Robbins advocates many of the things we are including in this book, like sufficient sleep and exercise, as well as cutting out smoking and excessive alcohol consumption, in order to help fuel our brains. As Tony Robbins (2019) says, *'The core benefit of eating right is having the energy to meet your dreams and lead a fulfilling lifestyle.'*

In our day-to-day work and general lifestyle, we place great demands on our brain to respond to various degrees of stimulation. We then wonder why overloading an undernourished brain can lead to mental fatigue, low mood and impaired cognitive functioning. I'm sure you see the theme here. This leads to reduced productivity.

WATER

We need water in order to survive. While Mahatma Gandhi survived 21 days without food, the longest humans can survive without water is around 100 hours depending on other factors like environmental temperature (Kottusch et al, 2009). When researching the importance of water for our productivity, I found that most articles cite Mitchell and colleagues who as far back as 1945 wrote that the human brain and heart is composed of 73 per cent water, with the lungs being 83 per cent water, the skin 64 per cent water, the muscles and kidneys 79 per cent water and the bones 31 per cent water. When the body does not have enough water, we become dehydrated; signs include feeling thirsty, tired, headachy or dizzy and our urine output decreasing, which can lead to kidney failure. Sometimes I forget to drink when engrossed in what I am doing, but I can always tell when I am feeling dehydrated. I get tired and my thinking becomes scattered and erratic. I literally can't think or see straight.

Water is needed for a variety of reasons. It helps to keep our body temperature regulated and without it we become dehydrated. Even small amounts of dehydration can cause low mood, reduce concentration and increase headaches (Armstrong et al, 2012). Positively, water can boost your mood and energy levels and can help reduce feelings of anxiety. It is also important as it helps lubricate and cushion the body's joints, spinal cord and tissues, so reduces the risk of long-term chronic conditions like arthritis.

Have you ever tried speaking in front of a room full of people only to have your mouth go dry? You are likely to become dehydrated when in such a stressful situation because of elevated heart rate and heavier breathing. Also, being dehydrated can cause physical stress and therefore an increase in cortisol levels. This is as a consequence of the two-way relationship between stress and dehydration. It's a vicious cycle. Dehydration leads to stress and stress leads to dehydration.

Water also has a digestive function and helps the body produce saliva, which in turn helps break down food when we eat and also keeps our mouths healthy. We need water to enable our kidneys to work properly. The kidneys are a bit like a water filter: they filter the body's impurities which we excrete by way of urinating. When we don't urinate enough, it can lead to an accumulation of waste; this can lead to the formation of kidney stones, which are said to be very painful.

Although a diet including plentiful roughage, in the form of a balance of fruit and veggies, eaten alongside regular exercise, can keep our bowels healthy, we also need water to 'keep things moving', as it were. If we don't get it, we can become constipated. Constipation is dry, hard and compacted waste in our colon that is difficult to eliminate. One study conducted by Neri et al (2014) showed a loss in productivity and a need for medical intervention due to workers having constipation. So, don't pooh-pooh the idea of constipation!

HOW MUCH WATER IS ENOUGH?

Men generally require three litres of water a day, while women require two litres a day. One cup of water equates to about eight ounces of fluid. So, ideally, you need to be drinking between eight and ten cups a day (Simson, 2018).

Drink more water

- Water is a healthy and cheap choice for satisfying your thirst any time of the day or night.
- It also aids the absorption of vitamins and minerals and carries much-needed nutrients and blood around the body.
- If the idea of drinking plain water doesn't appeal, why not add fruit, vegetables or herbs to your water to add natural flavour.
- You could leave fruity herbal teas to cool and use this as a form of flavoured water.
- Plain tea, fruit tea and coffee (without added sugar) can also be healthy.

But watch out!

Diet drinks are high in artificial sweeteners, and likewise so-called fruit juices can be full of refined sugars as well as the natural sugars you'd expect.

Lisa's top tips

One of my favourite ways of drinking more is to take approximately 2.5cm of raw ginger root, chop it and blend it (skin and all), put it into a large jug and top up with hot water, leaving it to infuse. You can also add lemon, honey, or even cinnamon for a 'hug in a mug'. The resulting drink is very good for your respiratory system and comforting especially in the winter. I always try to keep a bottle of water on my desk. Every few minutes I take a mouthful, and I find a mouthful every few minutes soon adds up to a cup over the hour.

SUGAR

Experts believe sugar is just as addictive as cocaine. The addiction is fuelled by the release of dopamine, a neurotransmitter that helps you feel a pleasurable 'high' in a similar way to drugs like cocaine. That's why eating sugar can make us feel good (Rada et al, 2005). The downside is that the reward centre in the brain is trained to crave sugar and we become addicted to it, or rather to the pleasurable feeling it gives us, so end up wanting more. Addiction is the compelling need to repeat an activity or ingest a substance that we know is harmful to us, but since it makes us feel good, we keep ingesting it.

Sugar tastes nice and gives us that short, sharp energy boost we sometimes crave. But we then get an energy slump about 20 minutes later which drives us to have more sugar in order to replicate the energy rush we enjoyed earlier. Except one doughnut is no longer enough, we need two to get the same rush, then three and so on. In order to keep feeling good, we need to increase the amount of sugar we eat as well as the frequency, despite the side effects of headaches, weight gain and hormone imbalances. These are classic behaviour traits of someone who abuses substances (Avena et al, 2008; Nestler, 2005).

While I'm sitting at my computer typing up a support plan, munching on a biscuit or two and slurping my coffee, grabbing the telephone to deal with yet another query, I'm eating in an absent-minded way. Half an hour later I wonder why I'm hungry, so end up rooting through my drawers to see what else I have hidden to give me another quick fix. Vasselli et al (2013) explain a high intake of sugar, such as biscuits, fizzy pop and cakes, can over time lead to our bodies becoming resistant to the hormone leptin. Leptin tells the body it's had enough to eat. Resistance to leptin can be one of the reasons why we may never feel full. So, we eat more than we should, we gain weight, we experience low mood and increased anxiety, and this results in reduced productivity.

ALCOHOL

Our relationship with alcohol, personally and as a society, is a complex subject. My focus here is only going to be on how the effects on the body impact our productivity.

Water in centuries gone, before suitable sanitation, was always considered to be unsafe. Fermentation processes converted sugar found in fruits or grains to ethyl alcohol and carbon dioxide, producing alcoholic drinks which, at the time, were a safer way to stay hydrated as the brewing process killed any harmful bacteria. I don't drink much alcohol, but I'm not opposed to the occasional gin and tonic. I actually quite like the fuzzy feeling it creates as my bloodstream carries alcohol up to the brain, I just don't like the impaired judgement that comes with it: *'Alcohol is not the answer, it just makes you forget the question'* (author unknown).

As soon as you take your first sip of alcohol it takes around ten minutes for you to begin to feel its effects as it enters the bloodstream via the stomach and small intestine. Alcohol is then carried around all the organs in the body. After an hour the brain is affected, concentration is reduced, judgement becomes impaired and retention of information is prevented, resulting in memory loss. We've all experienced a great night out, after which we know we enjoyed it but we can't remember most of it!

The World Health Organization (2018) explains that alcohol is *'a psychoactive substance with dependence-producing properties that has been widely used in many cultures for centuries. The harmful use of alcohol causes a large disease, social and economic burden in societies.'*

I know anecdotally that many professionals use alcohol as a means of unwinding after a hard day at the office. But the next morning, feeling dehydrated and hungover can lead to reduced concentration, poor decision making, judgement errors and poor quality of work. It can also impact upon your working relationships if colleagues have to cover your work at short notice if you need to take time off to recover from excessive intake!

While we have already covered sleep elsewhere in the book, I do feel it is important enough to repeat that alcohol can reduce your ability for restorative, deep sleep. Cutting out the 'night cap' is one of the best ways you can improve your sleep. Getting a good night's rest allows you to be more alert and 'on point' the next day, so increases your ability to be more productive.

The Chief Medical Officer's guidelines for both men and women advise no more than 14 units a week spread out over several days (Department of Health, 2016). But it is easy to drink more units than you realise, so why not find out more via Drink Aware and Alcohol Change UK (see 'Useful Links' at the end of the chapter), which have lots of useful guidance and advice about alcohol, tracking the amount you drink and how to drink more responsibly.

CAFFEINE

Walker (2018) describes society's obsession with coffee (and therefore caffeine) as the largest unsupervised drug-related social experiment ever undertaken. While I may not indulge too much in drinking alcohol, coffee is another matter. Until I've had that first cup in the morning, you'd do well not to talk to me, or even look at me, or you risk such a withering look it's likely to turn you to stone. After my first cup my brain feels like it's been jump started the way you would do with a car battery that's just died.

> *After water, coffee is the most popular beverage worldwide, with people drinking approximately 1.6 billion cups a day.*
> (Cappelletti et al, 2015)

Caffeine is dissolved into the bloodstream and is taken to the brain where it functions in the same way as adenosine. Adenosine is a molecule that binds to receptors in the brain, with the effect of slowing down nerve cell activity, causing drowsiness. Adenosine is instrumental in helping us get to sleep. Caffeine binds to the adenosine receptors, stopping the adenosine from doing its job, and speeds up nerve cell activity, thus promoting alertness.

At the same time, this triggers the pituitary gland to believe this sudden increased brain activity is occurring for some imminent emergency and sets off a hormonal chain of events to enable adrenaline, the 'fight or flight' hormone, to be released. Just by having a large cup of coffee, our airways open up, we have increased blood flow to muscles which tighten in readiness for action, our blood pressure rises and the liver releases sugar into the bloodstream for extra energy.

Your liver also produces an enzyme that removes the caffeine from your blood and once it has successfully removed it, you will experience the 'caffeine crash'. This is because while you are enjoying the 'benefits' of the caffeine the adenosine in your brain continues to build up, waiting to seize an opportunity to take back control of your brain – and when it does the feeling is overwhelming (Walker, 2018).

Fatigue sets in which in turn makes us crave the mid-morning and mid-afternoon caffeine fuel injection to set off the same chemical chain of events to boost our alertness once again. While we may benefit in the short term from caffeine-induced alertness, it's no fun at 3am, when you find yourself wide awake pondering life's great questions such as *'Why is the sky blue?'* or *'Do penguins have knees?'* An early evening coffee can lead to significant levels of caffeine still being present in your body hours later and can impact on your ability to sleep. When you do eventually fall asleep, you are likely to wake up groggy, which leads to another hit of caffeine to boost your alertness and thus the cycle repeats.

Caffeine is addictive. If you've ever tried going without it you will have experienced some unpleasant symptoms. Caffeine withdrawal begins anywhere from 12 to 24 hours after your final cup. If we stop ingesting caffeine, blood vessels widen and blood flow is increased to the brain, initially causing headaches which settle once the brain adapts to the increased blood flow (Merideth et al, 2009). Reducing your caffeine intake to one or two cups a day and having a 'no caffeine after lunch' approach can give you the benefits of caffeine without some of the problems. Be aware there's lots of hidden caffeine in carbonated drinks. There's caffeine in regular tea and green tea and 'decaf' versions of drinks are not completely caffeine free.

CONCLUSION

What struck me when researching this chapter is the vast amount of information out there about nutrition. It really is a minefield, especially when there are daily reports contradicting what is good for us and what is not. It seems like we no sooner get our heads around what we should be eating and drinking than a new piece of research turns that upside down.

My view is everything in moderation. We know what we should be doing – for example, eating at least five portions of fruit and vegetables and drinking two litres of water a day. Simply getting on and doing it is the biggest issue for me, and I'm sure I'm not alone. But we need to get it right because good nutrition is not just for our physical health, but also for our mental and emotional health, and it can help manage our stress and aid our productivity.

NUTRITION CHECKLIST

Start with:

- eating a healthy balanced diet;
- limiting processed foods (including takeaways);
- eating more fruit and vegetables;
- limiting your sugar intake;
- considering your caffeine intake;
- being alcohol sensible;
- drinking more water;
- maintaining a weight that's right for you.

Then try:

- introducing prebiotics and probiotics into your diet;
- being more mindful of your emotions and the connection to food;
- combining good nutrition and exercise;
- ensuring a good night's sleep;
- and drinking even more water!

USEFUL LINKS

During my research I found these following links really useful and hope you do too:

Alcohol Change UK https://alcoholchange.org.uk/

Blood Pressure UK www.bloodpressureuk.org/Home

British Association of Dieticians www.bda.uk.com/

British Nutrition Foundation www.nutrition.org.uk/

Clean Eating www.dummies.com/food-drink/special-diets/eating-clean-for-dummies-cheat-sheet/

Drink Aware www.drinkaware.co.uk/

Eatwell Guide www.gov.uk/government/publications/the-eatwell-guide

Food Allergy and Deficiency Testing www.eye-on-health.co.uk/cms/home

Food and Mood www.mind.org.uk/media/34727115/food-and-mood-2017-pdf-version.pdf

Health of the Nation Strategy http://navigator.health.org.uk/content/health-nation-%E2%80%93-strategy-health-england-white-paper-was-published

Heart UK www.heartuk.org.uk/

Holistic Wellness Project www.holisticwellnessproject.com

Live Well www.nhs.uk/livewell/healthy-eating/Pages/Healthyeating.aspx

Promoting Health and Well-being https://publichealthmatters.blog.gov.uk/2015/12/30/promoting-health-and-wellbeing-nationally-a-year-in-review/

Why Eat a Balanced Diet? www.eatbalanced.com/why-eat-balanced/

REFERENCES

Anderson, T and Yeo, G (2019) *It Takes Guts: Introduction to Gut Health*. Audible Podcast. [online] Available at: www.audible.co.uk/pd/It-Takes-Guts-Introduction-to-Gut-Health-Audiobook/B07JZD5HFD (accessed 12 February 2020).

Armstrong, L E, Ganio, M S, Casa, D J, Lee E C, McDermott, B P, Klau, J F, Jimenez, L, Le Bellego, L, Chevillotte, E and Lieberman, H R (2012) Mild Dehydration Affects Mood in Healthy Young Women. *Journal of Nutrition*, 142(2): 382–8.

Avena, N M, Rada, R and Bartley G (2008) Evidence for Sugar Addiction: Behavioral and Neurochemical Effects of Intermittent, Excessive Sugar Intake. *Neuroscience & Biobehavioral Reviews*, 32(1): 20–39.

BNF (British Nutrition Foundation) (2018) Protein. [online] Available at: www.nutrition.org.uk/nutritionscience/nutrients-food-and-ingredients/protein.html?limitstart=0 (accessed 28 December 2019).

Bravo, J A, Forsythe, P, Chew, M V, Escaravage, E, Savignac, H M, Dinan, T G, Bienenstock, J and Cryan, J F (2011) Ingestion of Lactobacillus Strain Regulates Emotional Behavior and Central GABA Receptor Expression in a Mouse via the Vagus Nerve. *Proceedings of the National Academy of Science of the USA*, 108(38):16050–5.

Cappelletti, S, Daria, P, Sani, G and Aromatario, M R (2015) Caffeine: Cognitive and Physical Performance Enhancer or Psychoactive Drug? *Current Neuropharmacology*, 13(1): 71–88.

Cho, Y and Kim, J (2015) Effect of Probiotics on Blood Lipid Concentrations: A Meta-analysis of Randomized Controlled Trials. *Medicine*, 94(43). [online] Available at: https://www.ncbi.nlm.nih.gov/pmc/articles/PMC4985374/pdf/medi-94-e1714.pdf (accessed 25 February 2020).

Cornah, D (2006) Feeding Minds: The Impact of Food on Mental Health. [online] Available at: www.mentalhealth.org.nz/assets/ResourceFinder/Feeding-Minds.pdf (accessed 4 February 2020).

Cryan, J (2019) in Anderson, T and Yeo, G *It Takes Guts: Introduction to Gut Health*. Audible Podcast. [online] Available at: www.audible.co.uk/pd/It-Takes-Guts-Introduction-to-Gut-Health-Audiobook/B07JZD5HFD (accessed 12 February 2020).

Cryan, J F and Dinan, T G (2012) Mind-altering Microorganisms: The Impact of the Gut Microbiota on Brain and Behaviour. *Nature Reviews (Neuroscience)*, 13(10): 701–12.

Department of Health (2016) UK Chief Medical Officers' Alcohol Guidelines Review: Summary of the Proposed New Guidelines. [online] Available at: https://assets.publishing.service.gov.uk/government/uploads/system/uploads/attachment_data/file/489795/summary.pdf (accessed 4 February 2020).

Emeran, A, Mayer, E A, Tillisch, K and Gupta, A (2015) Gut/Brain Axis and the Microbiota. *Journal of Clinical Investigation*, 125(3): 926–38.

Enders, G (2015) *Gut: The Inside Story of Our Body's Most Underrated Organ*. London: Scribe.

Fenton, K (2017) Health Matters: Obesity and the Food Environment. [online] Available at: https://publichealthmatters.blog.gov.uk/2017/03/31/health-matters-obesity-and-the-food-environment/ (accessed 28 December 2019).

Friedman, R (2014) What You Eat Affects Your Productivity. [online] Available at: https://hbr.org/2014/10/what-you-eat-affects-your-productivity (accessed 4 February 2020).

Fukuda, S, Toh, H, Hase, K, Oshima, K, Nakanishi, Y, Yoshimura, K, Tobe, T, Clarke, J M, Topping, D L, Suzuki, T, Taylor, T D, Itoh, K, Kikuchi, J, Morita, H, Hattori, M and Ohno, H (2011) Bifidobacteria Can Protect from Enteropathogenic Infection through Production of Acetate. *Nature*, 469(7331): 543–7.

Heart UK (nd) Saturated Fat. [online] Available at: www.heartuk.org.uk/low-cholesterol-foods/saturated-fat (accessed 28 December 2019).

Hemarajata, P and Versalovic, J (2013) Effects of Probiotics on Gut Microbiota: Mechanisms of Intestinal Immunomodulation and Neuromodulation. *Therapeutic Advances in Gastroenterology*, 6(1): 39–51.

HumanN (2019) Protein Deficiency: Signs, Symptoms, and Recommendations. *HumanN*. [online] Available at: https://www.humann.com/nutrition/protein-deficiency/ (accessed 25 February 2020).

Kang, E J, Kim, S Y, Hwang, I H and Ji, Y J (2013) The Effect of Probiotics on Prevention of Common Cold: A Meta-analysis of Randomized Controlled Trial Studies. *Korean Journal of Family Medicine*, 34(1): 2–10.

Kelly, J R, Kennedy, P J, Cryan, J F, Dinan, T G, Clarke, G and Hyland, N P (2015) Breaking Down the Barriers: the Gut Microbiome, Intestinal Permeability and Stress-related Psychiatric Disorders. *Frontiers in Cellular Neuroscience*, 9: 392.

Klarer, M, Arnold, M, Günther, L, Winter, C, Langhans, W and Meyer, U (2014) Gut Vagal Afferents Differentially Modulate Innate Anxiety and Learned Fear. *Journal of Neuroscience*, 34(21): 7067–76.

Kottusch, P, Tillmann, M and Püschel, K (2009) Survival Time without Food and Drink. *Archiv fur Kriminologie*, 224(5–6): 184–91.

Lamprecht, M, Bogner, S, Schippinger, G, Steinbauer, K, Fankhauser, F, Hallstroem, S, Schuetz, B and Greilberger, J F (2012) Probiotic Supplementation Affects Markers of Intestinal Barrier, Oxidation, and Inflammation in Trained Men: A Randomized, Double-blinded, Placebo-controlled Trial. *Journal of International Social Sports Nutrition*, 9(1): 45.

McDonald, M (2017) Nutrition and Mental Health: Obvious, yet Under-recognised. [online] Available at: www.mentalhealth.org.uk/blog/nutrition-and-mental-health-obvious-yet-under-recognised (accessed 4 February 2020).

mentalhealth.org.uk (2017) Diet and Mental Health. [online] Available at: www.mentalhealth.org.uk/a-to-z/d/diet-and-mental-health (accessed 4 February 2020).

Merideth, A, Addicott, L, Yang, A M, Peiffer, L R, Burnett, J H, Burdette, M Y, Chen, S H, Kraft, R A, Maldjian, J A and Laurientia, P J (2009) The Effect of Daily Caffeine Use on Cerebral Blood Flow: How Much Caffeine Can We Tolerate? *Human Brain Mapping*, 30(10): 3102–14.

Merrill, R M (2012) Presenteeism According to Healthy Behaviours, Physical Health, and Work Environment. *Popular Health Management*, 15(5): 293–301.

Mitchell, H H, Hamilton, T S, Steggerda, F R and Bean, W H (1945) The Chemical Composition of the Adult Human Body and Its Bearing on the Biochemistry of Growth. *Journal of Biological Chemistry*. [online] Available at: www.jbc.org/content/158/3/625.short (accessed 4 February 2020).

Neri, L, Basilisco, G, Corazziari, E, Stanghellini, V, Bassotti, G, Bellini, M, Perelli, I and Cuomo, R (2014) Constipation Severity Is Associated with Productivity Losses and Healthcare Utilization in Patients with Chronic Constipation. *United European Gastroenterology Journal*, 2(2): 138–47.

Nestler, E J (2005) The Neurobiology of Cocaine Addiction. *Science & Practice Perspectives*, 3(1): 4–10. [online] Available at: www.ncbi.nlm.nih.gov/pmc/articles/PMC2851032/ (accessed 4 February 2020).

NHS (2017a) Fat: The Facts. [online] Available at: www.nhs.uk/live-well/eat-well/different-fats-nutrition/ (accessed 28 December 2019).

NHS (2017b) Overview: Vitamins and Minerals. [online] Available at: www.nhs.uk/conditions/vitamins-and-minerals/ (accessed 28 December 2019).

NHS (2018a) Leaky Gut Syndrome. [online] Available at: www.nhs.uk/conditions/leaky-gut-syndrome/ (accessed 28 December 2019).

NHS (2018b) The Truth about Carbs. [online] Available at: www.nhs.uk/live-well/healthy-weight/why-we-need-to-eat-carbs/ (accessed 28 December 2019).

Peterson, J B (2018) *12 Rules for Life: An Antidote for Chaos*. Toronto: Random House.

Rada, P, Avena, N M and Hoebel, B G (2005) Daily Bingeing on Sugar Repeatedly Releases Dopamine in the Accumbens Shell. *Neuroscience*, 134(3): 737–44.

RCP (Royal College of Psychiatrists) (2015) Eating Well and Mental Health. [online] Available at: www.rcpsych. ac.uk/healthadvice/problemsdisorders/eatingwellandmentalhealth.aspx (accessed 4 February 2020).

Ríos-Covián, D, Ruas-Madiedo, P, Margolles, A, Gueimonde, M, De Los Reyes-Gavilán, C G and Salazar, N (2016) Intestinal Short Chain Fatty Acids and Their Link with Diet and Human Health. *Frontiers in Microbiology*, 7: 185.

Robbins, T (2019) 5 Ways To Fuel Your Brain. [online] Available at: www.tonyrobbins.com/health-vitality/5-ways-to-fuel-your-brain/ (accessed 4 February 2020).

Rooks, M G and Garrett, W S (2016) Gut Microbiota, Metabolites and Host Immunity. *Nature Reviews (Immunology)*, 16(6): 341–52.

Segain, J, De La Bletiere, D R, Bourreille, A, Leray, V, Gervois, N, Rosales, C, Ferrier, L, Bonnet, C, Blottiere, H and Galmiche, J (2000) Butyrate Inhibits Inflammatory Responses through Nfkb Inhibition: Implications For Crohn's Disease. *Gut*, 47(3): 397–403.

Sender, R, Fuchs, S and Milo, R (2016) Revised Estimates for the Number of Human and Bacteria Cells in the Body. *PLoS Biology* (2016) 14(8): e1002533.

Simson, R (2018) 10 Healthy Ways to Increase Your Fluid Intake. [online] Available at: www.roswellpark.org/cancertalk/201805/10-healthy-ways-increase-your-fluid-intake (accessed 4 February 2020).

Sinn, D H, Song, J H, Kim, H J, Lee, J H, Son, H J, Chang, D K, Kim, Y H, Kim, J J, Rhee, J C and Rhee, P L (2008) Therapeutic Effect of Lactobacillus Acidophilus-SDC 2012, 2013 in Patients with Irritable Bowel Syndrome. *Digestive Diseases and Sciences*, 53(10): 2714–18.

Talbott, S (2007) *The Cortisol Connection: Why Stress Makes You Fat and Ruins Your Health, and What You Can Do About It* (2nd ed). Alameda, CA: Hunter House.

Vasselli, J R, Scarpace, P J, Harris, R B and Banks, W A (2013) Dietary Components in the Development of Leptin Resistance. *Advances in Nutrition*, 4(2): 164–75.

Walker, M (2018) *Why We Sleep*. London: Penguin Random House.

Waterfall, T (2018) The Scientific Link Between Healthy Eating and Productivity. [online] Available at: www.managers.org.uk/insights/news/2018/august/the-scientific-link-between-healthy-eating-and-productivity (accessed 4 February 2020).

World Health Organization (2018) Alcohol – Key Facts. [online] Available at: www.who.int/news-room/fact-sheets/detail/alcohol (accessed 4 February 2020).

Yurcheshen, M, Seehuus, M and Pigeon, W (2015) Updates on Nutraceutical Sleep Therapeutics and Investigational Research. *Evidenced-based Complementary and Alternative Medicine*. doi: 10.1155/2015/105256.

Exercise: how moving more means you do more

Stephen

INTRODUCTION

I hated physical education (PE) at school. It was all muddy cross country and team sports that I really wasn't very good at. I loved cycling. I had a Grifter. Grifters were cool. This was the 1980s and everyone that was anyone had a Chopper. Except those who were even cooler than those that had a Chopper. They had a Grifter. I had a Grifter. Looking back now (you can find a few pictures on the internet, and I found one for sale on eBay) it was very much the forerunner of the mountain bike in its style. Very cool. But still, I hated PE.

When I talk to people about exercise this is a familiar story. For many of us, our relationship with exercise, like our relationship with food, can be a complicated one and is often rooted in our past. When it comes to doing what is good for us, we often know what to do but have difficulty doing it. Engaging in exercise relies on motivation which is often lacking at the end of a busy day. It also relies on setting realistic goals. This chapter is not about becoming a marathon runner, or someone who is in the gym at 6am every morning, but rather is about sustaining a level of physical activity that promotes well-being. Because being well promotes positive feelings which in turn promote productivity.

WHAT DO WE MEAN BY EXERCISE AND HOW MUCH SHOULD WE DO?

Cairney et al (2014) point out that really 'exercise' is a subset of physical activity. We are physically active in many more ways than when we are 'exercising'. The terms physical activity and exercise are generally used interchangeably which creates a feeling that things like washing the car, tending the garden and hanging out the washing don't count towards our goal of being physically active. They do. Physical activity does not need to take place in a gym or in a track suit, although it's not a problem when it does, and such exercise is also very good for us. Chatterjee (2018) suggests that one of the problems with our relationship with exercise and food is that the diet industry has turned these things into a simple equation of calories in and calories out. This misses the point that the human body is a complex 'machine' and therefore all of the things we are talking about in this book have a complex interaction with each other. Move around more and eat well and things will largely take care of themselves, he says.

Making a start is the hardest part. Burkeman (2019) explains this by observing what is probably familiar to many of us. We set ourselves up to engage with a new task because we know it's going to be good for us. We become excited at the prospect of positive change but then another part of us rises up like an uninvited guest whom we forgot to inform about the impending change, hell bent on upending our plans, often with success. We'll look at some tips later in the chapter on how to approach exercise to help you engage.

The UK Chief Medical Officer's *Physical Activity Guidelines* (2019) are in line with general advice that has been given for some time. As adults we should aim for 150 minutes of moderate exercise, or 75 minutes of vigorous exercise, per week. They define moderate exercise as breathing a little faster but being able to sustain a conversation and vigorous exercise as breathing fast with some difficulty maintaining a conversation. Assuming you're not a fan of the vigorous end of the scale then you are aiming for just over 20 minutes of gentle exercise per day as a base line. The Chief Medical Officer also suggests some strength training twice a week. That sounds very achievable to me. The benefits stated in the guidelines are many and centre mainly on physical health; they point out, for example, that such a level of exercise can reduce your chance of developing type 2 diabetes by 40 per cent, cardiovascular disease by 35 per cent, joint and back pain by 35 per cent and cancers (noting particularly colon and breast) by 20 per cent. I find those statistics quite exciting and a good return on 20 minutes of moderate exercise per day. Also, engaging in this level of exercise reduces the risk of depression by 25 per cent, manages stress and improves sleep. The officer's advice, succinctly put, is '*Some is good, more is better*' (2019, p 35).

THE PSYCHOLOGICAL REWARDS

Exercise can be a gateway habit that leads us to apply ourselves effectively to other areas. As any sports person will attest, engaging in physical activity is hard work. It makes you feel uncomfortable, sometimes a little, sometimes a lot. You will get sweaty and flushed and your muscles will probably ache afterwards. Cairney et al (2014) tell us that those who endorse exercise as a means of coping with the rigours of life are also more likely to endorse, and engage in, other positive behaviours. Self-application in deliberately engaging in something uncomfortable helps us cope with 'discomfort' when found in other areas. This has a positive impact on our productivity as, when things are difficult and there's a lot to do, deliberately setting our intention to the task is helpful. If we build the habit of being able to do this through exercise, then it will permeate into other areas of our lives.

Szabo et al (2013) say that the positive impact of exercise is immediate and is evident after just one session. They state that it is a valid non-pharmaceutical intervention for stress and mood disorder that goes hand in hand with the other physical health benefits. They go on to say that self-selected exercise at an intensity that the person is comfortable with triggers a positive impact on well-being. They report that even ten minutes of engagement in exercise is sufficient to experience psychological benefit. I have always felt that small changes accumulate into large impacts and this appears to be so in terms of exercise. Jackson (2013) talks about breaking the government's suggestion of about 20 minutes a day down into two 10- to 15-minute sessions, one before work and one during lunchtime, to give a boost and combat stress throughout the day. Where fatigue is also an issue, engaging in short bursts rather than sustained exercise can be helpful as it may be easier to motivate yourself to do this rather than be confronted with trying to undertake 30 minutes or more in one go.

Working towards and achieving a physical goal triggers psychological rewards – the power of small wins that I explore in the productivity chapter. This fuels a 'can do', optimistic approach to other life tasks. Optimism is an effective tool when trying to cope with life's ups and downs (Cairney et al, 2014). I'm reminded of a story I read in a blog many years ago where the writer wanted to motivate himself to get fit but kept failing to engage. So, he set himself the target of doing just one press up a day. He got up in the morning and got down on the floor and did his one press up. He then thought, '*Well, while I'm down here I might as well do another*'. He never just did one press up. He set a target that was achievable, that motivated him, rather than something that felt too grand. Sometimes we set ourselves goals that merely get in the way rather than motivate us. Interestingly Szabo et al (2013) also found that fitness levels were not particularly relevant to positive outcomes. They reported that individuals who were used to fitness training and those who were not both saw a mood enhancement of around 50 per cent after exercising.

THE IMPACT OF STRESS ON MOTIVATION TO EXERCISE

One of the problems with initiating engagement in exercise is that motivation can be at a low ebb when you feel stressed. If you are having trouble fitting everything into your packed schedule already, how do you then fit exercise in? In an American study led by Matthew Burg of Yale University in 2017 they explored the relationship between stress and exercise (Burg et al, 2017). They observed that engagement in a healthy active lifestyle can be elusive for many and that experiencing stress can be a barrier to maintaining good health. They pointed to studies that had shown that levels of stress in individuals can predict low levels of physical activity. This is a 'double bind' because, as we shall see, exercise can mitigate stress. Stress stops you exercising yet exercise improves your response to stress.

As we have already seen (Chapter 3), stress can produce a fight or flight response that is driven by the production of adrenaline and cortisol. This response is designed to urge you into the physical response that was required for our ancient ancestors to run away from danger and find safety. Often in our modern world the ability to 'run away' from the stress while sat at the computer screen or in a meeting is not available to us. But the chemical response still takes place and significant levels of these things in our bodies are not good for us.

Burg et al (2017) wanted to check whether the experience of stress did indeed impede engaging in physical activity. They recruited just over 60 generally healthy adults who reported limited engagement in exercise. They measured their physical activity levels objectively through the use of a Fitbit and subjectively through daily questions about their anticipated stress and exercise levels and their actual levels. At the start of the day they asked them if they expected the day to be stressful and whether they were likely to exercise. At the end of the day they asked them how stressful their day had been and whether they had exercised for 30 minutes or more. What they found was that a 30-minute bout of exercise had benefitted some in relation to the stress they were feeling but had had no impact on others. For some it had increased their stress. They identified that anticipating a stressful day correlated with a lower likelihood of exercise but also that engaging in exercise was a predictor of lower stress levels at the end of the day. They had shown the bi-directional nature of the relationship between stress and exercise.

I would hypothesise that those who found that exercising increased stress may well have been those who struggled to find time to fit it in. In our deliberations about being productive, what we know is that there is a relationship between all the elements we are exploring. Being organised is crucial to how you approach the things that you need to do and the things that would be beneficial to do. It doesn't surprise me to find that this study identifies that viewing your day as being stressful leads to low engagement in exercise. I'd argue that viewing your day in this way leads to low engagement in everything you try to do. Stress and disarray are the fuel of procrastination, and the two often go hand in hand. You need to be organised to be effective.

Self-efficacy is the ability to find it in yourself to move to action in order to deal with the situations that present themselves and is important in engagement with any of the activities of life. It is the internal belief in oneself to be up to, and able to get on with, the task at hand (Bandura, 1982). As with the relationship between stress and exercise, there is a circular relationship between self-efficacy and exercise. If you lack confidence in your ability or have a poor self-image then maybe you don't want to present yourself in public exercising. I have struggled for years in gym spaces, feeling inadequate comparing myself to others, feeling everyone is looking at me. They are probably not, but when that's how it feels it provides an obstacle that gets in the way of us engaging. As my favourite philosophers the Stoics argue, 'the obstacle is the way'. We must find a way through it. Overcoming such obstacles builds our confidence and we then become more effective.

THE INTEGRATION OF STUDIO CYCLING INTO A WORKSITE STRESS MANAGEMENT PROGRAMME

Clark et al (2014) explored how an exercise programme could improve confidence and stress management. They facilitated a 12-week stationary bike programme in a workplace setting that also included some coaching around stress management.

They discovered that participants reported being more confident in areas of their lives beyond exercise.

Many people had reported before the programme that stress had led them to make poor food choices but that, after the programme, they were more confident in their ability to select healthy options.

They noted 'significant and clinically meaningful improvements in perceived stress, current stress level and confidence for managing stress. Participants also reported having improved physical activity level, perceived health, spiritual well-being, sleep, support for maintaining healthy living, nutrition and quality of life' (Clark et al, 2014, p 171).

The study effectively shows the relationship between all the self-care elements we are discussing and adds weight to the idea that exercise is a gateway activity to improvements in many spheres of our lives.

WHAT DOES THE SCIENCE SAY?

Engaging in exercise promotes blood flow to the brain, providing more oxygen which in turn promotes cognition. It promotes increases in endorphins and serotonin which have been linked to psychological well-being. Endorphins trigger a positive feeling in the body due to their pain-relieving properties and could possibly be part of the euphoric feeling that people describe after engaging in exercise – the 'runner's high' as it is sometimes called. Jackson (2013) states that being physically active enhances how the body handles stress through changes in the response of our hormones to stress. Szabo et al (2013) feel that there are too many competing factors to show a direct causal relationship, but this chemical increase is definitely a factor. Serotonin is sometimes referred to as the happy chemical because of its positive impact on mood, with low levels being shown to be present in people experiencing depression and anxiety. These chemical mechanisms can account for the positive psychological effects of exercise on well-being, but they are not the full story. It is possible that exercise simply serves as a break from the stress-inducing elements of our lives, giving us time to create psychological 'space' (Jackson, 2013). It is likely to be a combination of these factors that helps us.

LUNCH BREAK ANYONE?

One of the problems associated with people instigating engagement in physical activity stems from practitioners often placing the cause of stress in the workplace but placing the solution outside of the workplace (Marc and Osvat, 2013). This means they don't prioritise physical activity (or possibly any self-care) while at work. This is seen most in the ineffective use of breaks. In fact, I think I'm safe to say that a 'working through your lunch break' culture permeates many modern organisations, including social work settings. A study at Bristol University (Coulson et al, 2008) showed that exercise during a lunch break boosted mood and motivation by 41 per cent and improved the ability to deal with stress by 20 per cent. Those are much needed boosts. Using exercise as a positive distraction was also reported as reducing stress and anxiety by Cairney et al (2014).

De Bloom et al (2017) explain that there are two elements to recovery from job stress. The first is a reduction of demands, which is often outside of our control. The second is engaging in pleasurable activities, of which exercise can be one. The lunch break and some gentle exercise can establish a perceived restoration of the self and enhance mental resources to take into the afternoon. Puig-Ribera et al (2017) noted a reduction in stress as a consequence of a 'sit less, move more' programme they initiated as part of their research. They showed that a lunch break and walk improved staff retention and sickness and led to more mindful practice. De Bloom et al (2017) point to numerous studies that show engaging in a leisure activity you enjoy brings long-lasting changes to the body, which has benefits for psychological health. While such engagement requires effort, the benefits are clear.

THEORIES AND MODELS ACCOUNTING FOR THE PSYCHOLOGICAL BENEFITS OF EXERCISE

The sympathetic arousal hypothesis

Regular exercise improves fitness, which can result in a decreased resting heart rate. Heart rate can provide a rough measure of sympathetic arousal, with sympathetic arousal being associated with our fight or flight response to stress. Exercise improves cardiovascular health, achieving a lower resting heart rate, lower sympathetic activity (exercise 'burns off' stress hormones) and lower arousal at rest. This promotes relaxation and tranquillity.

The cognitive appraisal hypothesis

This hypothesis suggests that people engage in exercise to 'escape' psychologically from stress. The engagement in exercise promotes psychological relief so the person continues to exercise. If the person stops exercising, they experience a withdrawal state characterised by sluggishness and irritability so return to exercise to escape those feelings, so maintaining their motivation to exercise.

The affect regulation hypothesis

This hypothesis proposes a dual effect on mood. It firstly produces a positive psychological state of longer duration than momentary emotions we might feel and, secondly, decreases negative feelings, therefore improving mood.

The thermogenic regulation hypothesis

This idea relies on a mind–body loop where a relaxed body promotes a relaxed mind. Exercise increases body temperature, creating a relaxed state similar, for example, to a warm bath or a sunny day, and therefore reduces negative feelings.

The catecholamine hypothesis

Catecholamines are involved in the stress response and have been found in increased levels after exercise. They are involved in regulating mood and are known to be important in problems like depression. It is not clear whether changes in catecholamines throughout the body have an effect on brain catecholamines as it is impossible to measure them in the human brain.

The endorphin hypothesis

This is the 'runner's high' phenomenon. The idea is that exercise results in increased levels of endorphins in the brain giving a euphoric feeling. Runners report a pleasant sensation of well-being and a sense of achievement, creating positive feelings that, in the short term at least, mask fatigue and the pain of strenuous exercise.

Adapted from Szabo et al (2013)

WHAT SORT OF EXERCISE WORKS?

The guidance from the Chief Medical Officer in the UK (2019) is that you should engage in three sorts of exercise: cardiovascular (exercise that gets you out of breath), strength (exercise that involves some sort of resistance) and stretching and balance (exercise that improves flexibility and core strength). Chatterjee (2018, p 152) says simply that '*the world is your gym*'. You don't need fancy equipment or a gym membership to do enough of what you need to do to improve your well-being and productivity by improving your fitness.

Cardiovascular activity

Cardiovascular activity is any physical activity that increases your breathing and your heart rate, generally uses your major muscle groups, and often uses all of them. Running, walking, swimming and cycling all fit into this category. One activity you could consider to get you started is simply walking. It requires no specialist equipment, just a comfortable pair of shoes. The idea of trying to take 10,000 steps a day seems to have resonance in the public conscience and is a really simple thing to aim for. The number 10,000 isn't particularly special in any way. It feels like a good psychological number to me. For most people it probably represents more steps than they would usually take in a day, so it encourages you to do that little bit more. Most smartphones or cheap step-counting devices would count your steps for you if you wanted to keep track.

Equally, lots of routine activities may give you a low level of cardiovascular activity. Walking from the car into work (you could park a little further away), gardening, washing the car, taking the stairs, doing housework, or, instead of picking up the phone, standing up and walking to your colleague's office to talk to them. There's a double bonus with the last one as interaction also helps to promote well-being – so that's a win–win.

You can also do a cardio workout routine at home by combining exercises that leave you breathless. You need very little space and some fairly basic workout clothing like shorts, t-shirt and some suitable shoes. A search of the internet turns up many short workouts that will show you what to do, from simple five-minute sequences to longer, more intense ones. They include exercises you may well be familiar with like star jumps, lunges, running on the spot and burpees (my personal fitness nemesis).

Remember, the recommendation is to do a minimum of 20 minutes per day of this type of activity. More is good.

There are many great initiatives to get you up and moving.

Couch to 5k

This NHS-backed training plan is excellent. It gets you exercising three times a week and starts with alternating walking and running to get you to the goal over nine weeks of being able to run 5km without stopping. That would be a great achievement.

It emphasises rest days which are so important no matter how fit you are.

There's even an app.

Find out about it here: www.nhs.uk/live-well/exercise/couch-to-5k-week-by-week/

Parkrun

Once you can run 5km (or even if you need to walk some of it), you could find a local Parkrun. I can honestly say that doing Parkrun has kept me on track with at least getting some exercise every week when busy or lacking motivation. The fact you exercise with other like-minded people is the key here.

Parkrun was founded by Paul Sinton-Hewitt in 2004 at Bushy Park in London and has really taken hold, with runs taking place every Saturday morning at 9am across the world. There are almost 700 in the UK.

Parkrun is a measured and timed 5km course. You need to go to the Parkrun website and register and print off a barcode. They scan this at the end of the run and that means they can work out your time which they'll email and text to you. And it's all free. Check out the website to find one near you. I have always found the people at Parkrun to be friendly and supportive of those new to running or new to a particular location. Give it a try!

Find out more here: www.parkrun.org.uk/

Strength building activities

The recommendation of the Chief Medical Officer is that we engage in strength training twice a week. There are many types of strength training, but it usually involves some form of resistance or the moving of a heavy object. That heavy object could be you! When you think of strength training you probably conjure up pictures of weightlifting or weight machines in the gym. You can, though, in your own home, engage in strength training that uses just your own body weight. Exercises such as push ups, squats, plank and calf raises are all good. There is some cross over between strength building exercises and cardiovascular exercises. I can guarantee you that when I do push ups and squats my heart rate rises. You will find that engaging in one engages you in the other a lot of the time. Exercises like burpees and lunges (which are predominantly cardio) are also using your body weight, building strength and getting you out of breath.

Stretching and balance activities

There has been a surge in interest in the last decade or so in activities like yoga and tai chi. They often combine elements of exercise with mindfulness or meditation, which is a great combination. It has been shown that a 60- to 90-minute session of either of these activities, performed two or three times a week, can reduce stress and improve feelings of well-being. Even shorter sessions can be effective. Fifteen minutes of chair-based yoga has been shown to have a positive psychological impact on levels of stress and a physiological impact on respiration and heart rate (Jackson, 2013). We know that stress elevates both of these things, so engaging in yoga briefly at your desk, and maybe some mindful breathing, could have an impact that may benefit you. There are many articles on the internet that explore this, and you can find them by simply searching for 'yoga at your desk'. There are also many online videos or classes at your local sports centre to support you with this.

LET'S GET STARTED

Before you start any exercise programme, and particularly if you have not exercised before, you should consider whether you need to take advice from your doctor. If you have any health conditions that may be limiting or have experienced any problems like dizziness, chest pain, joint problems or light headedness, then it would be advisable to be checked over physically and be offered specific advice by your doctor. In making suggestions regarding exercise, a book like this can only ever offer general information. So, consider if you need to take personal guidance. If you start exercising and feel dizziness, faintness, pain or shortness of breath then stop immediately. The often-stated mantra 'no pain no gain' is simply not true. Exercise should be and can be a pleasurable activity, particularly at the levels we have seen are required to promote psychological well-being and enhance productivity.

WALK BEFORE YOU RUN – LITERALLY AND METAPHORICALLY

The one sure-fire way of not maintaining any sort of positive relationship with exercise is to do too much, and particularly too much too soon. At the risk of repeating myself, small changes lead to big outcomes. This is the case with all self-care, not just exercise. The cumulative effect of lots of small changes can be huge. Haruki Murakami (2009, p 71) describes this phenomenon in his delightful running memoir *What I Talk About When I Talk About Running*, when he says, *muscles are like work animals that are quick on the uptake. If you carefully increase the load, step by step, they learn to take it. As long as you explain your expectations to them by actually showing them examples of the amount of work they have to endure, your muscles will comply and gradually get stronger.*

The key words here are 'carefully increase' and 'gradually'.

The important thing is to set yourself a realistic goal. You may well have heard the acronym SMART before. If you make a goal SMART it helps you see progress. SMART goals are:

- **S**pecific;
- **M**easurable;
- **A**ttainable;
- **R**elevant;
- **T**ime limited.

With the Chief Medical Officer's guidance in mind you might decide to walk three times during the week for 20 minutes with a longer walk of an hour during the weekend when you have more time. That's 120 minutes. Not quite the 150 minutes recommended, but if you've not exercised before then that's ok, you can build up to 150. You'll do this for four weeks and see how you are getting on.

This is Specific. It can't be any clearer really – a specific exercise for a specific length of time. It's Measurable. Did you walk for the time you aimed for? It's Attainable. I think it is. You have more time on a weekend, hence the longer walk, and you are not walking every day so that you can recover in case you have any muscle soreness. Muscle soreness is inevitable when you exercise and should disappear after two or three days. If it doesn't, consult your doctor. It is Relevant. We know what the advantages of doing this are. They are both physical and psychological. In a demanding profession we need to build our physical and psychological resilience and we have seen how exercise helps this. Finally, it's Time limited. You are going to do this for four weeks and see how you are getting on. You're then going to set yourself another goal.

There is a range of opinion about how long it takes to build a habit, but certainly few people advocate that it takes anything less than a month. If you can do this for a month then there's a good chance you will have built an exercise habit. Building this habit relies on the release of the dopamine and endorphins that we discussed earlier. These chemicals give us the feel-good factor, that 'runner's high', that will hopefully drive us to do more. When you're ready, you can move on to other goals and incorporate the other types of exercise that are recommended, such as strength training, stretching and exercises that improve balance. The same rules apply. Start small and build up.

DO WHAT YOU LOVE

As well as running at school, which I later came to love, we played football, cricket and rugby. As one of the less sporty pupils I found this quite stressful, as I don't like to let people down, so as the ball came towards me I would become anxious, which would lead to me fumbling the kick or the catch which fuelled feelings of inadequacy. This is not what we want. What we want is for you to find a physical activity that you love to do. If you find something you love to do, you are more likely to stick at it. Wulf et al (2014) discovered that when people were shown a range of exercises and self-selected the ones that they did, they did more repetitions of the exercises than others who had been prescribed their exercises by another person.

The good news is there are so many things you can engage in. We've already talked about walking, which surely has to be the most accessible way to exercise. Open your door and go! There are lots of things you can do in your home with online videos or DVDs to guide you. For a relatively small cost you can invest in your health with some light weights, running shoes, resistance bands... the list is vast. Despite what I've already said about exercise having the potential to be a no, or low, cost activity, I have to advocate for your local gym or even personal trainers. While this can be expensive, particularly the latter, it can pay dividends. Certainly, if you are going to buy weights, or other equipment, to use at home it would be worth paying for someone who is qualified to show you how to use them. Not only to avoid injury but also because, by using the equipment correctly, you will get more benefit. Good 'form', the way you do the exercise, is important in getting the most out of what you do. There is a huge range of exercise classes, from stationary bikes (often called 'spinning'), to high-intensity interval training and functional training, which uses exercises that mimic activities we would do in our daily lives to improve our general functioning. These things are useful but not essential. You can be active enough to promote well-being without spending anything.

FIND AN EXERCISE BUDDY

Rackow et al (2015) found there were many benefits to turning exercise into a social activity. Exercising with a supportive friend was found to improve self-efficacy (the ability to motivate oneself to action). They also showed that planning exercise and setting goals with someone else improved engagement. The exchanges between exercise partners also helped to monitor how things were going towards achieving goals, through giving effective feedback. Effective feedback can be a significant motivating factor. They also found that the emotional support and encouragement from the partner improved self-efficacy. Jackson (2013, p 18) confirms this when she says that *'group exercise or encouraging stressed clients to find a workout partner is an excellent idea because it can provide a support network and accountability.'*

As well as all of this research information, it's just more fun! If you are walking or running and chatting as you go, the time and the miles fly by. Encouraging each other and telling each other how you are feeling when undertaking repetition-based exercises (weight training or body weight exercises) is also very motivating. I find having someone simply count the 'reps' with the odd word of encouragement in between helps massively. Also, exercising with a friend means you are more likely to engage as you won't want to let them down.

PENCIL IT IN

Committing to a specific plan has been found to improve goal attainment. We can use fancy words for it like externalising ideas or behaviour planning, but personally I prefer to simply call it 'writing it down'. Having a plan reduces thoughts about the as yet unachieved goal and also frees up mental resources for other tasks (Masicampo and Baumeister, 2011). The simple task of writing down what you are going to do commits you to it psychologically and putting it in your calendar allocates your time to the task.

FAIL TO PREPARE, PREPARE TO FAIL

Everything, and I mean everything, comes down to planning. To get the most out of all of the facets of your life you need to plan meticulously. A place for everything and everything in its place. Being properly prepared enhances your chances of success and makes starting something much easier. Avoiding procrastination is the key to achieving goals. In relation to exercise, check you have picked a suitable time when the chances of something getting in the way are at their lowest. Ask yourself if you have given yourself a big enough time slot? Give yourself more time than you think you will need. Have you got all of the things ready and available to you that you will need? If not, plan when you will make them ready, or go and get them now.

If I want to run first thing on a morning, at some point the night before I place my training shoes at the front door, I place my shorts and t-shirt at the end of the bed, and I set my alarm. When I get out of bed, I have my clothes and shoes on before I've even thought about it. I know from experience if I have to rifle through my drawers to find the specific shorts I want and my favourite t-shirt then I am likely to end up putting the kettle on and not bothering. If I'm going for a walk, I get my walking boots out of the shed, where they live, the day before, I check the weather, I print a route if I need one and I place them all to hand. I know… it might sound somewhat over the top, but I guarantee that it means, more often than not, I end up doing the thing that I've planned and, importantly, it ends up being an enjoyable success. If we enjoy things we are more likely to do them again.

Plan it, do it.

CONCLUSION

In a Canadian study (Cairney et al, 2014) 40 per cent of the people surveyed said they used exercise to cope with stress and the same people were more likely to endorse other positive strategies for coping. They were also less likely to use alcohol as a 'self-care' strategy. Exercise, it would seem, *is* a gateway habit. The researchers noted that exercise reduces tension, promotes relaxation and provides an effective way to cope with stress. In terms of coping with the rigours of a complex work environment they also noted improvements in feelings of self-worth and personal control, both of which are important when exposed to stressful situations. They considered exercise to be a 'win–win' strategy as it can help us cope with the stress we have already experienced and be a preventative measure to mitigate stress that we may experience in the future. It gives us a physical resilience and emotional control in the difficult situations that we often are faced with as practitioners.

The benefits are clear. One single session of aerobic exercise improves mental functioning and performance, giving us faster processing, faster reaction times, a clear head and better short-term memory performance. This leads to more effective planning.

In terms of your physical well-being your weight may drop. While the focus on exercise here is about productivity, losing a little weight if you need to isn't a bad thing as being overweight increases your chances of some health conditions which in turn could impact negatively on your productivity.

Exercise will certainly increase your stamina, not just when exercising, but also when engaging in a mentally demanding profession. You will have a renewed vigour as a consequence of those 'happy' chemicals coursing through your body and you will get a sense of achievement from all of your 'small wins' that you will take into other areas of your productive life.

Szabo et al (2013) found that both running and meditation promoted positive changes in mood. This really comes as no surprise to me. The physical, mental and emotional aspects of our 'self' are so interlinked. I see running or walking as meditation (or mindfulness) in motion. When simply putting one foot in front of the other and engaging mentally with how your body feels you can switch off to the other things that are going on in your life. Haruki Murakami, who we met a few paragraphs ago, says, '*I just run. I run in a void. Or maybe I should put it another way: I run in order to acquire a void. But as you might expect, an occasional thought will slip into this void*' (2009, p 17). I'd argue for letting in those things that encroach. When trying to deal with a difficult conundrum I find running helps me focus exclusively, in a mindful way, on whatever it is that I need to consider while placing all other things out of my head. As a social worker I have solved some of the most difficult things circulating in my head while out for a run.

Engaging in exercise, as with any other self-care activity, is not easy. We need to be prepared. We need to find the time. The irony with exercise is that it improves the areas of our life that get in the way of exercising. We've seen how stress leads to a lack of motivation and how a lack of confidence leads to not engaging. If we do engage, though, stress is reduced and we feel more confident. When we were in the midst of a difficult situation, one of my managers when I was a social worker used to say, '*We need to get in front of this*'. This is true of exercise. The benefits are such that we need to push past the feelings that stop us and experience what it has to offer. We have seen how engaging in exercise can give you 'time out' from everything else. Exercise and meditation create a mind–body loop where each element looks after the other. As you are probably already seeing, all of the elements of self-care we are considering have their role to play in creating well-being. All have their role to play in terms of our productivity. If we are feeling energetic, have control of our emotions and have created the habit of easily initiating action, then we will be more productive in all areas of our lives.

REFERENCES

Bandura, A (1982) Self-efficacy Mechanism in Human Agency. *American Psychologist*, 37(2): 122–47.

Burg, M M, Schwartz, J E, Kronish, I M, Diaz, K M, Alcantara, C, Duer-Hefele, J and Davidson, K W (2017) Does Stress Result in You Exercising Less? Or Does Exercising Result in You Being Less Stressed? Or Is It Both? Testing the Bi-directional Stress-Exercise Association at the Group and Person (N of 1) Level. *Annals of Behavioral Medicine*, 51(6): 799–809.

Burkeman, O (2019) Your Shadow Self. *New Philosopher*, 24(May–July): 27–8.

Cairney, J, Kwan, M Y W, Veldhuizen, S and Faulkner, G E J (2014) Who Uses Exercise as a Coping Strategy for Stress? Results from a National Survey of Canadians. *Journal of Physical Activity and Health*, 11(5): 908–16.

Chatterjee, R (2018) *The 4 Pillar Plan*. London: Penguin Random House.

Chief Medical Officer (2019) *UK Chief Medical Officers' Physical Activity Guidelines*. London: Department of Health and Social Care.

Clark, M M, Soyring, J E, Jenkins, S, Daniel, D C, Berkland, B E, Werneburg, B L, Hagen, P T, Lopez-Jimenez, F, Warren, B A and Olsen, K D (2014) The Integration of Studio Cycling into a Worksite Stress Management Programme. *Stress Health*, 30(2): 166–76.

Coulson, J C, Mckenna, J and Field, M (2008) Exercising at Work and Self-reported Work Performance. *International Journal of Workplace Health Management*, 1: 176–97.

De Bloom, J, Sianoja, M, Korpela, K, Tuomisto, M, Lilja, A, Geurts S and Kinnunen, U (2017) Effects of Park Walks and Relaxation Exercises during Lunch Breaks on Recovery from Job Stress: Two Randomized Controlled Trials. *Journal of Environmental Psychology*, 51(August): 14–30.

Jackson, E M (2013) Stress Relief: The Role of Exercise in Stress Management. *American College of Sports Medicine Health and Fitness Journal*, 17(3): 14–19.

Marc, C and Osvat, C (2013) Stress and Burnout among Social Workers. *Social Work Review / Revista de Asistenţă Socială*, 12(3): 121–30.

Masicampo, E J and Baumeister, R F (2011) Consider It Done! Plan Making Can Eliminate the Cognitive Effects of Unfulfilled Goals. *Journal of Personality and Social Psychology*, 101(4): 667–83.

Murakami, H (2009) *What I Talk About When I Talk About Running*. London: Vintage.

Puig-Ribera, A, Bort-Roig, J, Giné-Garriga, M, González-Suárez, A M, Martínez-Lemos, I, Fortuño, J, Martori, J C, Muñoz-Ortiz, L, Milà, R, Gilson, N D and McKenna, J (2017) Impact of a Workplace 'Sit Less, Move More' Program on Efficiency-related Outcomes of Office Employees. *BMC Public Health*, 17: 455. doi:10.1186/s12889-017-4367-8.

Rackow, P, Scholz, U and Hornung, R (2015) Received Social Support and Exercising: An Intervention Study to Test the Enabling Hypothesis. *British Journal of Health Psychology*, 20(4): 763–76.

Szabo, A, Griffiths, M D and Demetrovics, Z (2013) Psychology and Exercise. In Bagchi, D, Nair, S and Sen, C K (eds) *Nutrition and Enhanced Sports Performance, Muscle Building, Endurance, and Strength* (pp 65–74). London: Academic Press.

Wulf, G, Heidi, E F and Tandy, R D (2014) Choosing to Exercise More: Small Choices Increase Exercise Engagement. *Psychology of Sport and Exercise*, 15(3): 268–71.

5 Mind full or mindful: giving yourself space

Lisa

INTRODUCTION

To truly appreciate the context of this chapter, I would recommend you read my story at the beginning of the book. But if, like me, you prefer to dip in and out of chapters, I will give you a brief summary. I'm a social worker. It took a long time for me to realise this is something 'I do' rather than something 'I am'. When I first qualified, I believed I could fix the world. When the world was not being fixed, I became very disillusioned. '*Surely if I am good at what I do*', I thought, '*then why isn't the world being fixed?*' Then one day the penny finally dropped. For all my good intentions and goodwill, I was never going to fix the world. The reason being, the world is full of people who simply don't want to be saved or fixed. Once I realised this, it enabled me to understand that my disillusionment with the profession came down to me. My attitude towards the profession changed, from what I personally felt it should be, to what it actually is. Talk about a lightbulb moment!

During the first seven years of my career I 'crashed and burned' several times. How? I simply never learned the lesson that it was my attitude to social work that was the problem. I continued to work in exactly the same way as I mentioned in my biography at the start of the book. Whenever I was not physically at work, I was mentally at work, every minute of every day. Thinking, thinking and thinking. I literally could not switch off. So, what did I do to change?

This chapter is going to be a little different from the rest of the book, which focuses upon the steps we can take in order to increase our productivity by practising self-care. I am going to slow down a little, take a more scenic and spiritual route, if you will. This route, in essence, will show you how to practise self-love and in turn, as a natural by-product, self-care will be easier, and this will allow for increased productivity! So, grab a cup of green tea, light some incense, curl up on the settee with a cosy blanket, play some soothing background music and relax, as you read on.

SPIRITUALITY

What do I mean by being spiritual? The natural starting point here is to ask, what does this mean to you?

- Take a few minutes to reflect upon what being spiritual means to you.
- You may even find it useful to jot some thoughts down on a piece of paper to help organise your thinking.

If you need something to get you going, think about this: '*spirituality… the human quest for personal meaning and mutually fulfilling relationships among people, the nonhuman environment, and, for some, god*' (Canda, 1988, p 243).

In truth, I don't think there is a right or wrong answer. Your spirituality is how you define it. Everyone is different. Everyone has their own culture, beliefs and truths, so what you may feel is right for you will be different to someone else. When you take a moment to think about it, spirituality could be more about having a belief system that exists outside our socially constructed selves, a connection to something larger than our individual self, or a search for the greater meaning of life. Something that connects us all maybe. My personal belief is we all come from the same source, God, but in truth religion and spirituality are totally different things. Religion is very much a collective, an ideology with a specific doctrine underpinning a dogma which unites people of similar beliefs around the world. By contrast, spirituality is about *you*. It's about you as an individual, having your own experience and connecting with yourself and other people and, for some, God. As Deepak Chopra states, '*Religion is a belief in someone else's experience. Spirituality is having your own experience*' (quoted in Garrett, 2016, p 18).

Like life, being spiritual is fluid, so there will be times in your life when it flows easily without thinking and other times when you feel challenged. When you are riding this particular wave, all the self-care tips, on resilience, good nutrition, quality sleep and exercise, may well be looking after your physical and mental well-being, but on an emotional and spiritual level, the scales can be well and truly unbalanced.

When spending time reflecting as I went through what I refer to as my 'storm of despair', I realised part of my problem was caring. I cared about my clients, their families, my colleagues and friends. One of the things I failed to even consider was that before I could begin to care for others, I needed to care for me first. I thought I was failing in my career. My spiritual growth had collapsed, and I was in the midst of the greatest storm of my life. It was then that I turned to mindfulness, meditation, energy healing and self-forgiveness. It is these things that have helped heal and soothe my soul, repair that has helped move me from despair. What was storm is now calm as I have slowly learned that '*you can't pour from an empty cup*'.

THE COGNITIVE TRIANGLE

Albert Ellis (1994) explains how assumptions we have about ourselves and our external world serve to guide us throughout our life and in turn influence how we react to any situation we happen to encounter. I'm confident you will have heard about cognitive behavioural therapy (CBT), which, as McLeod (2019) explains, is a talking therapy based on the assumption that abnormal behaviour can be traced back to irrational thinking and built, partially, on the back of Ellis' ideas around these assumptions about ourselves.

Gross (2015, pp 796, 797) explains how Arron Beck takes this further by focusing upon what he calls a negative cognitive triangle, primarily developed around a person's self-belief when diagnosed with depression (LoudLizard, nd). It explores three elements: the self, the world or environment, and the future.

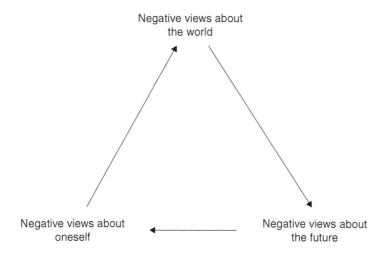

If we take a moment to look at the diagram, we can see how negative views about our-selves can influence how we view the world around us and how we view our future. It is a concept that plays an integral part in Beck's treatment of negative automatic thoughts (TNAT) for depression frequently used in CBT. When considering this model in relation to my own experiences, I can totally identify with the principles. The way I viewed my role as a social worker influenced my self-worth (the self), especially when I felt I was not really helping people around me in the way I felt they should be helped (the world) and this made me become extremely disillusioned with my future within social work (the future).

Imagine, before leaving home to go to work this morning, you have an argument with your spouse, or the children. They aren't ready on time, making you leave later than normal, and you get behind schedule. The traffic getting to work is gridlocked and you hit every red light in the city. As a result, you arrive 20 minutes late for an appointment with a client.

Take a moment to consider the cognitive triangle.

Think about:

- Self – how does this situation make you feel about yourself?
- World/environment – how does this situation make you feel about your family, your clients, your employer, your external world in general?
- Future – how does the above influence your hopes and fears for the future?

How does all of this influence your behaviour when you are having to explain to your client why you are late?

Can you see how sometimes things are just beyond your control?

When we are sitting with a client, colleague, friend or family member, our conscious self, our thinking mind, enables us to listen to what is being said. Our professional training around communication skills, learning to hear what is not being said, and observing body language, it all stems from the ego. The ego helps us to perceive our external world, adapt to our given reality and solve problems, as well as memorise information and produce ideas. It is our conscious self, the thinking mind, the ultimate and most primitive function of which is to keep us safe from harm (Gross, 2015). It always amuses me how my mind works. I view the 'fight or flight' response we have talked about throughout this book as being the 'rough and ready' format for keeping me safe. While these primal survival tools are useful to us, the problem is that what we 'think' can end up controlling how we 'feel' and this can then influence our 'actions', which, as we have seen, is the principle of Beck's cognitive triangle.

MINDFULNESS

I suspect most people these days will have heard of mindfulness, but not necessarily know what it is other than perhaps it being the latest fad! Truth be told, it has been around forever! The word mindfulness suggests it has some relation to our minds, our thinking and our cognitive processes. While not exactly the same, I identify it as a distant cousin of CBT. Baer (2003) describes mindfulness as being attentive to one's present moment, to the here and now, without actually judging it. Kabat-Zinn (2013) also explains how mindfulness is a useful psychological process that enables you to become aware of your current experience or situation, and to be in the present moment, but not judge yourself within that moment.

Thinking back to our earlier task, you could argue your mind was full of things you know you needed to do for your family, work, clients and where you needed to be. If we were to take a mindful approach to being late, we would simply take a moment to acknowledge there was a catalogue of incidents that had contributed to our running late that morning, as well as us not being organised enough to set off to work that bit sooner. Being mindful allows us to understand that sometimes this is just how life goes. Sometimes things are simply beyond our control. The more we dwell on them, the more we become mentally unfocused, and this can reduce our productivity. Being mindful helps you to understand this. It makes you stop, take a breath and examine how any given situation is making you feel at any given moment in time. It allows you to pause the cognitive triad roundabout in order for you to recognise, then start to understand, how *you* can be your own worst enemy. Once you start to recognise any potentially destructive patterns of behaviour, it allows you to become more empowered to change these for the better and this will help you to manage your stress and anxiety, which in turn increases productivity.

True mindfulness is not the quick fix we all want in this fast-paced, hectic world of ours, and that's one of the reasons why some people dismiss it as being unhelpful. But if you stick with it, you truly do change the way you view life, and when you view your life differently, your life can change for the better.

Reiki principles by Dr Mikao Usui

Just for today…

I will not worry.
I will not get angry.
I will be honest.
I will count my blessings.
I will give love and show respect for every living thing.

Origins of mindfulness

There remain varying views about the origins of mindfulness, but it is generally said to have its roots in the Buddhist concept of observing your thoughts and actions. Vetter (1988) explains how Buddhism is more a practice of inner reflection than an actual religion. It is the art of getting to know yourself and developing a deeper understanding of who you are. It is about reaching down into the parts of yourself that you know need to change, observing how the change arises and how you follow through with this change. Brian Heater (2017) explains how when we practise mindfulness we move from our heads, always thinking and judging, to our hearts, where we feel more. It allows us to become more in tune with our intuition. We develop compassion – not just for other people, but for ourselves. We become kinder to ourselves, and we begin to understand and love ourselves more, allowing ourselves to become humble, and less defensive and selfish. We feel peaceful because we are no longer battling with ourselves and no longer dwelling on others who aim to do battle with us. I know from personal experience the process of reaching inside yourself can trigger painful but often necessary changes. I stuck with it and came out the other side, a stronger, wiser, kinder and humbler person. Without going through all that I did, I would not be in the position I am in now, able to share my story in the hope it will be helpful to you should you be in the midst of your storm. For that reason alone I am thankful.

Awareness

Being mindful is about the connection between your thoughts and feelings at any given moment, being aware of both your internal and your external world. Tasha Eurich (2018) explains that internal self-awareness is about how we identify with our values, our dreams, aspirations, thoughts, feelings, strengths and weaknesses and how these all impact upon the people around us. Self-awareness is about recognising what is going on around us and how we react to it; for example, a client can say something in passing, which may suddenly trigger an emotion or lead us on a mental journey or to a memory that seems to rise up from nowhere. Very much in the same way, a song playing on the radio can trigger a happy or sad memory. We may not always be able to control the things going on around us, but we can control how we react to them or feel about them.

Take a few moments to think about something from your past that made you feel sad or angry. Remember the emotions from that time but do not dwell on them.

Notice how your physical body is responding to these memories and emotions *(I know my heart usually races, my stomach feels like it's in knots and I sweat, attractive!).*

Now bring your awareness back to the here and now. You may find it useful to make a few notes on your experience.

Do exactly the same thinking about a time when you were really happy *(I find myself smiling, which makes my eyes crinkle, I get a sense of serenity and I feel calm).*

Bring your awareness back to the here and now, again make a few notes on your experience.

What differences have you noticed in relation to how your physical body reacted just by you thinking about happy or sad memories?

Being non-judgemental

What do we mean by being judgemental? Rutter and Brown (2012) explain that being judgemental relates to forming a negative and critical opinion of others and is undesirable. I often hear people say that when we make judgements about others, we are actually making a statement about who we are rather than who they are. To quote Carl Jung, *'everything that irritates us about others can lead us to an understanding of ourselves'* (quoted in Woolfe, 2016).

Yet making judgements is something we do all the time. Gary McGee (nd) quotes Jiddu Krishnamurti: *'the ability to observe without evaluating is the highest form of intelligence'.* The underpinning reason why people judge can come down to a fear of failure, or other people not liking us, or abandonment and rejection. Judging others can help us feel better about ourselves, enable us to feel superior, but in reality it stems from ego (Gross, 2015), moving us, as social workers, away from the unconditional positive regard we should have towards others. Our minds can make snap judgements, automatic almost reflex-like assessments of what we perceive to be our reality at that moment. Daniel Kahneman (2011) refers to this in his book *Thinking, Fast and Slow*, where he talks about 'system one' and 'system two'. It is generally believed in the world of psychology that our thoughts can arise in two different ways, automatic thinking (system one) and deliberate thinking (system two). So, when you arrive late for your client's appointment because you slept in, or the rush hour traffic was a nightmare, and you may be thinking the day could not possibly get any worse, Kahneman (2011) might argue this is your 'system one' thinking. It's automatic, instant, intuitive, impressionistic and based upon irrational bias that leads you to jump to rash conclusions. If, on the other hand, you had taken a slower, more pragmatic 'system two' approach to thinking about what you needed to do today, planned ahead and been organised, the likelihood is you would have coped better with the delays. The problem is that if 'system two' were an animal, it would likely be a sloth, as it demands much slower, critical thinking, as well as time to do that thinking. That is why, when up against the clock, we often revert back to 'system one' thinking, that snappy, quick-fire kind of thinking related to our 'flight or fight' instinct.

Living in the present moment

Bil Keane (1994) states, '*yesterday is history. Tomorrow is a mystery; today is a gift, which is why we call it the present.*' Living in the present moment is just that: letting go of past experiences and not being overly consumed by something that may or may not happen in the future. We can get trapped in risk management by trying to anticipate something that has not happened yet, as a means of knowing what *could* happen and determining the necessary steps required to reduce the impact *if or when* it does (Taylor, 2017). Risk management demands we focus upon the future, yet mindfulness asks us to be in the present. This is one of the things I find the hardest about mindfulness, especially as I am still practising and have to manage risk on a daily basis!

Yet, truthfully, all we really have is the here and now. Not one of us is promised the next few moments in life. The past has gone, and the future has not yet occurred. Right here, right now, at this precise moment, you reading these words is the present moment. Eckhart Tolle in his book *The Power of Now* (Tolle, 2016), explains how the main cause of unhappiness is not any given situation, but your thoughts about the situation. He tells us that we have a choice and can decide what kind of relationship we have with the present moment. I think that is very powerful, and very much in keeping with our social work values around autonomy!

Our mind and thoughts are never still, they are always on the go. Our thoughts require energy, which is why when we overthink about things we end up feeling drained and exhausted. Being aware of this allows your focus to be more in this moment so you are not worrying about the past or the future. It allows anxious thoughts to disappear so you become less fearful of the future.

Mindfulness and social work

Nowadays with austerity and ever decreasing budgets, we, as social workers, need to be creative in our thinking in order to assist with problem solving. It's not just about thinking outside of the box but looking to see how we can get rid of the box altogether, as boxes cost money! Over time, our professional experience allows us to develop tried and tested suggestions to help others take control of their lives and become empowered. But this can mean we become too fixed or set in our ways of thinking, running the risk of prescribing one-size-fits-all solutions rather than being creative and person centred. Mindfulness, according to Siegal (2010), allows us to balance our emotions so we become more attuned to others, more flexible, and expand our insight into problems. This brings with it clarity and thus creative problem solving. Win–win.

As we've said before, sometimes our clients can say something to us that takes our attention in a different direction as our own thoughts, emotions and worries take over our thinking. Being mindful and aware of how a given situation is making you think or feel, allows you to connect more with your clients so you can gain a greater sense of understanding about what is going on in their lives, which in turn aids creative problem solving. When we do support someone to come up with their own solution as a result, we feel the power of that small win that Stephen talks about elsewhere in the book.

Malinowski and Lim (2015), when researching work-based mindfulness, found it led to non-reactivity and being non-judgemental (reduced system one thinking), which led to greater work engagement, increased job satisfaction and professional resilience in the work place. Another study showed participants following mindfulness training had greater working memory, focused attention, and reduced occupational stress and burnout at post-programme and follow-up (Roeser et al, 2013).

> I believe choosing to form a relationship with your present moment is one of the most spiritual aspects of self-care you can truly engage in. Why not try the following exercise.
>
> Close your eyes, take a long, slow breath in through your nose and slowly exhale through your mouth. Focus upon your breathing. Breathe in, breathe out.
>
> Take your awareness to your body. Notice areas that feel tense such as hunched shoulders. Are you frowning or clenching your jaw? If so, release the tension. Keep your focus on relaxing these parts for a few moments.
>
> Now do a small task (something like photocopying or washing up). Keep your attention and focus on the here and now during the task. Observe any thoughts that come to you but just let them go, don't hold on to or judge them.
>
> Notice how these thoughts are making you feel emotionally and how those emotions are affecting your body. Do this until the task is complete.
>
> How did that feel? Write down your thoughts.
>
> It is not that dissimilar to the task earlier in the chapter, but it is known as a waking meditation. Yes, you have just been meditating.

MEDITATION

One of the things I enjoy most about mindfulness is meditation. For years, like many people I'm sure, I viewed meditation as being something you did sitting cross-legged on top of a mountain, wearing a leotard, thumb and first finger touching, humming the sound 'om'. Have you ever sat on a bus or a train and allowed the movement and motion of the vehicle to rock you as you stare out of the window so your mind goes blank? A bit like daydreaming? Well, that is meditating. Meditation literally is a means of distracting your mind from the immediate world around you.

Origins

It is not really known for certain how or when meditation was first practised. The oldest documented evidence is wall art in the Indian subcontinent from approximately 5000 to 3500 years BCE showing people seated in a typical cross-legged posture (Everly and Lating, 2002). Meditation is believed to have been the fundamental practice in the earliest forms of Hindu schooling in India, while Chinese Taoist and Indian Buddhist traditions are said to have begun from the sixth to fourth centuries BCE. In the West, meditation is believed to have evolved with notable religious figures such as Philo of Alexandria (Jewish philosopher, around AD 1), the desert fathers of the Middle East (third century AD, Christian hermits living in the Scetis Desert of Egypt) and Saint Augustine, a Christian bishop (AD 354–430) (Yungen, 2006).

In Latin, *meditatum* comes from 'to ponder'; it forms the basis of the word meditation we know today. Whatever the origins, meditation is simply focusing your attention and allowing your mind to relax, just like staring out of a window while on the bus. There are various different types of meditation, but for now I am going to concentrate on Buddhist meditation as their practice fits beautifully with mindfulness, encouraging concentration to bring about clarity of thinking, a sense of calm and emotional positivity.

Buddhist meditation

To quote Timber Hawkeye (nd), author of *Buddhist Boot Camp*, '*stop trying to calm the storm, calm yourself and the storm will pass*'. Buddhists believe in 'right remembering', referring to this as '*sati*'. In 1881, Thomas William Rhys Davids first translated the Magadhan word *sati* (Middle Indo-Aryan liturgical language native to the Indian subcontinent) into its English meaning of mindfulness, referring to the activity of mind and constant presence of mind (Rhys Davids, 1881). It is this meditation technique that tends to be more popular in the West, helping us to understand more about how our minds work and what makes us 'tick'. When we link this knowledge about ourselves with understanding how our thoughts influence our emotions and behaviours, we can learn to overcome long-held coping strategies that prevent us from being productive and leading happy and fulfilling lives.

Mindful breathing

It may strike you how in the previous exercises we have focused firstly upon our breathing. This is known as mindful breathing, or, put simply, using the breath as a means of concentration. When you focus upon your breathing, it enables you to realise just how much your mind gets distracted all of the time.

THE POWER OF THREE

You can do the following breathing activity anytime and anywhere, even when standing in the queue at a supermarket checkout, en route to a client's house or before heading into court. And it's free!

Take a slow, steady, deep breath in through your nose for the count of three.

Hold this breath for the count of three.

Slowly exhale this breath out through your mouth for the count of three.

Repeat this three times or more if needed.

Sue Doucette (nd) explains that slow breathing activates the brain's hypothalamus, which is connected to the pituitary gland. They work in partnership to release neurohormones to prevent production and release of stress hormones, the result being the triggering of the body's relaxation response. In other words, when we breathe deeply, the brain receives a message to calm down and relax, which in turn sends a signal to the body to do the same. So, when we are in the heightened state of 'fight or flight', with adrenaline and cortisol whooshing around causing our heart rate to increase, our blood pressure to rise and our breathing to become faster, deep, focused breathing allows the body to lower its stress levels and reduce tension. Focused breathing makes the body think the moment of danger has passed and we can heave a sigh of relief. By concentrating on your breathing, you can become less restless, and it can help you to mentally reflect upon situations that would otherwise make you feel anxious and depressed. Imagine being able to reflect upon work in such a way that you can understand your words and actions without actually becoming emotionally drained and exhausted.

Steps to mindful meditation

Unlike Stephen, I have never run a marathon. I never run, and if ever you do see me run, you'd better run too as you can bet something is chasing me! I wouldn't even know where to start, yet I do know I would have to gradually increase my fitness, which takes time and practice. Meditation is the same. You can't expect to be able to sit for hours in a meditative state when you first start. Even after all these years of meditating, I still don't sit for hours.

All you need to do to make a start is take a few moments every day. Five to ten minutes a day can really make a difference. There are loads of short meditation videos on the internet which are great for getting you started. If you are wanting to build yourself up to sitting for longer, it may be useful for you to find a local meditation group. Again, the internet or social media can be useful to locate a group near to where you live or work.

Chris Bailey (2013) suggests the two things you need to get started are somewhere to sit and a timer, that's it! He also stresses that no matter where you sit, ensure your back remains straight, as this helps you to focus upon your breathing. I actually prefer to do my meditation as part of my night-time routine, so falling asleep is never a problem as I'm warm and comfortable. You can choose to invest in meditation benches or cushions, but equally you can sit upright on a dining chair. Most mobile phones these days have a timer on them, but again it is personal preference as to whether you want to purchase a timer.

I know when I talk about meditation, I get asked questions like '*What do you do with your hands?*' or '*Should I close my eyes?*' The beauty of meditation is, you make it your own! You do what is comfortable for you. Build up slowly and aim for ten minutes a day – more is better, but even five minutes a day is helpful.

One thing about meditation people can struggle with is what is known as the '*monkey mind*'. Richard Oldale (2018) explains how at times of quiet reflection, our mind can become mischievous, scattered and chattering, just like a monkey. When you try to breathe mindfully and clear your mind, you find various thoughts, cravings and even restlessness presenting themselves. Every time you catch sight of your monkey, or rather as soon as you realise your thoughts are wandering, Bailey (2013) recommends refocusing upon your breathing.

GUIDED RELAXATION

One of the things I often teach to students, friends, family or colleagues is guided relaxation.

Using the power of three breathing technique described earlier, get yourself comfortable and focus upon your breathing.

In a moment or two, allow your focus to move to your feet. How do they feel? Tight? Tense?

Purposefully allow them to relax, and as you do so, refocus upon your breathing.

In a moment or two, allow your focus to move to your calves. How do they feel? Tight? Tense?

Purposefully allow them to relax. Next, take your awareness to your knees. How do they feel? Relax them. Next your thighs, a few moments later all the way up your back, a few moments later your neck, then the top of your head, up and over towards your forehead, down to your cheeks, jaw and down to your stomach.

Now that every area of the body has been focused and relaxed, how do you feel?

What you should find as you do this exercise is that your breathing will have naturally slowed and become rhythmic by the time you have finished focusing upon relaxing each part of your body. With the whole of your body relaxed, it is a great way to help you relax enough to aid sleep, especially when the monkey mind just wants to talk about work! When I talk through this same guided relaxation with people, the response is usually '*Ahhhh, that was lovely, I feel so calm now.*' The next comment is usually *'Can you come and sit by my bed at night and talk me through this, as your voice is so calming?'* I often do this routine when trying to fall back to sleep after my usual night-time toilet visits. As soon as I am settling back down in bed, my body is, *'Right let's go back to sleep'*, but my mind ends up singing, *'Old MacDonald had a farm'*. The more you practise this relaxation the easier it becomes, I promise!

ENERGY

I said earlier, during my crash and burn, that one of the things I realised is how much I empathised with others. When we empathise with others, we are demonstrating our ability to place ourselves in the other person's shoes, to understand and feel what the other person is experiencing from within their frame of reference (Rothschild, 2006). What I never considered was, when doing so, we are exchanging so much of our energy with the person we are empathising with. By the very nature of the work we do as social workers, we do encounter some very dark and negative souls, spiritually speaking, who can, without realising, feed off our energy so much we end up with compassion fatigue.

What do I mean by energy?

In the nutritional chapter, we talk about the role vitamins and minerals play in helping the body to metabolise calories to expend energy. Yet energy is so much more. Taking a simplistic approach to physics, energy is vibrating molecules. Anything solid, even your kitchen table, contains molecules that vibrate and it's the same for us as humans (Sturdy, 2016). As humans we are walking, talking energy in the form of vibrating molecules. Without realising, it is thought we may pick up on other people's vibrational molecules, or rather their vibrational energy. Have you ever met someone for the first time and taken an instant liking to them? Have you ever been in a particular building or a house and felt either a good, or not so good, vibe? That, it's suggested, is vibrational energy.

Sharing energy

Years ago, I worked with someone who in many ways was lovely, but by the end of the day, I always felt so drained by them. They always made me feel as if they were sucking the energy from me. Dussault Runtagh (2012) explains that ill health can lower people's vibrational energy. The lower your vibrational frequency, the denser your overall energy becomes. When your energy is dense, it can impact upon your physical, mental and emotional well-being, so you may experience physical pain, discomfort and mental confusion and become more emotional. Bernstein (2012) helps us to understand how when people are hurting, they are focused upon what is going on in their world without realising their lowered vibrational energy can actually be quite toxic to others. By the nature of who we are, as empathic social workers, we can subconsciously absorb the anguish or anger of others and this can have a draining effect on us. You then go home at the end of the day still holding on to their negative feelings, which in essence you have claimed as your own.

Protecting our energy

So, what can we do to protect our energy, especially when we do need to be empathic in our work? Have you ever watched *Star Wars*? Now I'm not an expert on *Star Wars*, but I know they often activate an energy shield, which is a bit like a large, pearlised, opaque half bubble over a planet or a spaceship. This energy shield protects from enemy attack. Laser beams deflect off the energy bubble. I love this analogy as it is one of the simplest things I do to protect my energy. I visualise myself in a large bubble, which covers me from the top of my head to down under my feet. It expands outwards, literally wrapping around me like a cocoon. Why not try this the next time you find yourself with someone who is being really negative? The bubble will simply deflect their negativity and stop you absorbing their negative emotions. It doesn't matter what colour your bubble is, it doesn't even need to be a bubble. You can imagine being surrounded by mirrors, or putting a coat on and zipping it up, whatever works for you. Like anything spiritual, the intention behind the action is everything.

SELF-FORGIVENESS

The weak can never forgive. Forgiveness is an attribute of the strong.

Mahatma Gandhi

Despite knowing many simple techniques that I have learned during my spiritual journey, one of the things I have found the hardest is to forgive myself for being human. As social workers we can, and do, make mistakes. We can fall into the trap of wanting to 'fix' people, but in our desire to help we can sometimes place unreasonable and unachievable expectations on them. When we sit with clients we try to understand what life experiences they have been through, their social or cultural conditioning, and how this perhaps underpins their view of the world around them and in turn how that influences their actions.

What we fail to understand or even recognise is we often go through similar life experiences. We too have been socially and culturally conditioned and perhaps that skews our outlook on life. We, with the very best of intentions, then try to project our views and ideas onto them and when they aren't able to fulfil our expectations this can lead to us feeling like a failure. We haven't been able to help them as we wanted. We can feel disappointed that we haven't been the ones to help no matter how hard we have tried. We may feel we have let them down and have somehow failed as a social worker. That's often when my critical inner voice seems to thrive and come alive, whenever I make mistakes in any area of my life, particularly my working life. My inner voice tends to make nasty comments: '*Well you made a mess of that you stupid so and so*'. I would *never* dream of talking like that to someone else, but that's how I have talked to myself in times gone by. We don't realise now these self-depreciating comments hurt our inner self, that hidden, vulnerable part of ourselves we only reveal to our most trusted loved ones when we feel safe. It just takes a period of time in your life when you are already feeling vulnerable (for example a bereavement or a relationship breakdown) for this feeling of failure to become all consuming. This in turn can end up eating away at the very core of your humanity. We contemplate over and over why we couldn't help. All this musing can impact upon our sense of reasoning, and then our productivity reduces and our stress levels go up.

For all the benefits to our self-care discussed in this book – good nutrition, exercise, sleep, resilience – I believe one of the hardest things to do is simply be kind to ourselves. For years I have struggled with self-forgiveness and letting go of expectations of myself and others. This often leads to disappointment and hurt. Forgiveness is about engaging in a deliberate intention to release feelings of anger or bitterness you have toward an individual who has harmed you, regardless of whether they actually deserve your forgiveness (APA, 2006). Self-forgiveness is not about forgetting the wrong or even condoning it, but sits at the heart of helping you move on. The individual you may need to forgive may be you.

HO'OPONOPONO

As Maya Angelou said, *'Forgiveness is the greatest gift you can give yourself'* (cited by Shapiro, 2013). Self-forgiveness can be powerful. One technique I frequently use is the *Ho'oponopono* prayer. In Polynesian culture, holding onto anger and hurt is believed to be a cause of physical ill health (Oliver, 2002). I love the saying *'Holding onto anger is like drinking poison and expecting the other person to die'*, as it resonates with me. Matthew James (2010) explains how *Ho'oponopono* is a Hawaiian mantra, which enables the *letting go* of hurt in order to bring about forgiveness.

So how do we do it?

Well first of all you have to learn how to say it and, thankfully, the word *Ho'oponopono* is not the mantra! *'Ho'o'* means 'to make' and *'pono'* means 'right'. So *Ho'oponopono* literally means to *make–right–right*. It is the repetition of this prayer that gives the power to bring about forgiveness and in turn healing and letting go. In essence, *Ho'oponopono* takes us back to what we have explained earlier in this chapter. Our thoughts influence our feelings, which influence our actions.

The first step to *Ho'oponopono* is about understanding how *you* are responsible for everything in *your* mind. When a client 'off loads' their worries and hurt, this is brought into your awareness. To comprehend the enormity of what they are telling us, we end up internalising their anxiety and hurt. We empathise and absorb the other person's energy. This can resonate with that wounded part of our inner selves. We become sorry for them and can at times, depending upon how much their hurt resonates with us, end up grieving for them. Being mindful allows us to recognise how we feel hurt by others. Observing our thoughts and feelings but without actually judging or engaging with them, alongside using the *Ho'oponopono* prayer, can empower us to forgive ourselves for allowing ourselves to be hurt and to forgive those who hurt us.

HO'OPONOPONO PRAYER

There are four steps:

'I'm sorry.'
'Please forgive me.'
'Thank you.'
'I love you.'

Step 1: saying *'I'm sorry'*

When we make a mistake, all our clients want (sometimes!) is for us to admit the mistake and to apologise. We, in our inner self, are no different. Saying, *'I'm sorry'* out loud helps you to recognise how hurt you feel about whatever the situation or hurt might be.

Step 2: *'Please forgive me'*

When we ask for forgiveness, we are acknowledging the hurt. Once we acknowledge this, it makes it easier to let go of the negative feelings and thoughts attached to this hurt. If we think back to our scenario earlier in the chapter where we ran late for a client appointment, we can release the negative feelings attached to being late, just by apologising for being late.

Step 3: *'Thank you'*

I can probably count on the one hand the number of 'thank you' cards I have received in my social work career, so on the occasion when I do receive one I feel a real deep sense of gratitude. That one small gesture *really* does help me to appreciate what an important role I play in other people's lives, especially when I perhaps feel a little low and undervalued. It is this type of gratitude you need when thanking yourself or others with *Ho'oponopono*.

Step 4: the last step is about *love*

Take a moment to think of that special someone in your life, a parent, partner, child, or pet. What does that love feel like? Does it feel like a hug? Do you feel like you are cosy, wrapped in a snuggle blanket on a cold rainy, wintry day? The kind of love that makes you feel warm inside as if your heart is glowing. *'And in a sense, love is everything. It is the key to life, and its influences are those that move the world'* (Ralph Waldo Trine, cited in Parker, 2012). That is the feeling of love you need when telling yourself or others you love them with *Ho'oponopono*.

It really doesn't matter who or what you direct this mantra towards, be it yourself, another person or even a situation. The power of the prayer is very much about being genuine in your intention.

CONCLUSION

Returning to social work following my career break, I was apprehensive about the possibility of burnout. This was only natural as that is what led to my career break in the first instance. Yet 'back in the saddle' I am still standing strong. There are still days when I wonder why I do the job I do. I still have days of intense pressure and stress. My self-care practice means I mostly take the rough with the smooth and always *all in my stride.* I finally understand that social work – well, social work is just social work. As a friend once said to me, '*it is what it is*' and it doesn't necessarily mean it's you getting it wrong. The positive outcome of my crash and burn is that I returned to social work with a much more mature understanding of myself, both as an individual and as a practitioner.

I recognise and know my trigger points when I'm feeling close to the tipping point as my productivity reduces. I get tired, my thinking starts to become a little erratic, my gut feeling tells me I am physically starting to feel 'unsafe' in my practice, so I need to say '*no*' and that takes strength of character and courage. More importantly, I know when I need to disconnect and take time out for *me*.

Mine has been a *long*, rough and painful journey of self-discovery, but along the way, I have learned so much. Without these experiences I would never have been in the position I am today, sharing with you the importance of self-care and loving yourself. Give yourself permission to take a step back, rest when you need to. You are *not* being *selfish* but are taking care of you and your inner self.

Finally, I hope something within this chapter has resonated with you. Spirituality is a very personal thing, so I have made some practical suggestions below by way of a summary that should help you get started or continue with your spiritual journey.

Namaste – the spirit in me honours the spirit in you.

Start with...

Be mindful rather than having a mind full.
Practise meditation now and then, ideally at least once a week.
Breathe!
Relax.
Protect your energy.
Love and forgive yourself.

Then, think of the following...

Learn to understand what being spiritual means for you.
Live in the moment.
Recognise trigger points and stop judging yourself.
Stop criticising yourself and others.
Meditate as regularly as possible, even if for only a few minutes a day.
Remember your mindful breathing and relax.
Recognise who affects your energy.
Protect your energy every day.
Know you are only human and will make mistakes.
Forgive yourself for any mistakes you make.
Practice *Ho'oponopono*.
Love you for the simple reason that you are you!

USEFUL LINKS

During my research I found these resources really useful and informative.

Balance and Harmony, www.facebook.com/BalanceandHarmonywb/
Cassandra Sturdy's *The Twelve Attunements* (Sturdy, 2016), www.cassandrasturdy.com/
Chris Bailey's *Guide: Everything You Need to Start Meditating* (Bailey, 2013), https://alifeofproductivity.com/meditation-guide/
Eckhart Tolle, www.eckharttolle.com/
Go the Path Less Traveled, https://lonerwolf.com/
Headspace and meditation, www.headspace.com/science
Kate Jackson's article 'The Mindful Social Worker: How Mindfulness Can Help Social Workers Practice More Creatively' (Jackson, 2017), www.socialworktoday.com/archive/SO17p14.shtml
Michael Hammer, free music downloads www.michaelhammer.net/
Mind, www.mind.org.uk/
Mindfulness, www.mindfulnet.org/index.htm
Mindworks, https://mindworks.org/
Ronald K Bullis' *Spirituality in Social Work Practice* (Bullis, 1996)
Rudolf Steiner's *Theosophy* (Steiner, 1994), https://steiner.presswarehouse.com/sites/steiner/research/archive/theosophy/theosophy.pdf
Social work and mindfulness, www.communitycare.co.uk/2018/01/30/ofsted-praises-impact-mindfulness-course-retaining-social-workers/
Sue Doucette's 'Why Does Deep Breathing Calm You Down?' (Doucette, nd), www.livestrong.com/article/136646-why-does-deep-breathing-calm-you-down/
Talking Changes, www.talkingchanges.org.uk/
Tapping4Success, www.facebook.com/Tapping4success/
The spiritual journey is much like a winding path through a thick forest, https://lonerwolf.com/start-here/

REFERENCES

APA (American Psychological Association) (2006) Forgiveness: A Sampling of Research Results. [online] Originally available at: www.apa.org/international/resources/forgiveness.pdf (accessed 7 February 2009 and archived from the original PDF on 26 June 2011 at: https://web.archive.org/web/20110626153005/).

Baer, R (2003) Mindfulness Training as a Clinical Intervention: A Conceptual and Empirical Review. *Clinical Psychology: Science And Practice*, 10(2): 125–43.

Bailey, C (2013) Guide: Everything You Need to Start Meditating. [online] Available at: https://alifeofproductivity. com/meditation-guide/ (accessed 4 February 2020).

Bernstein, A (2012) *Emotional Vampires: Dealing with People Who Drain You Dry* (2nd ed). New York: McGraw-Hill.

Bullis, R K (1996) *Spirituality in Social Work Practice*. Washington, DC: Taylor and Francis.

Canda, E (1988) Spirituality, Religious Diversity, and Social Work Practice. *Social Casework*, 69(4): 238–47.

Doucette, S (nd) Why Does Deep Breathing Calm You Down? [online] Available at: www.livestrong.com/ article/136646-why-does-deep-breathing-calm-you-down/ (accessed 4 February 2020).

Dussault Runtagh, P (2012) The Benefits of Being in a Higher Vibration. [online] Available at: www.huffpost. com/entry/positive-energy_b_1715767 (accessed 4 February 2020).

Ellis, A (1994) *Reason and Emotion in Psychotherapy: Comprehensive Method of Treating Human Disturbances* (revised and updated). New York: Citadel Press.

Eurich, T (2018) *Insight: How to Succeed by Seeing Yourself Clearly*. London: Pan Macmillan.

Everly, G S and Lating, J M (2002) *A Clinical Guide to the Treatment of Human Stress Response* (2nd ed). New York: Kluwer Academic/Plenum Publishers.

Garrett, M J (2016) *Sacred Light: My Journey from Mormon to Mystic*. Bloomington, IN: Balboa Press.

Gross, R (2015) *Psychology: The Science of Mind and Behaviour* (7th ed). London: Hodder Education.

Hawkeye, T (nd) [online] Available at: https://quotecatalog.com/quote/timber-hawkeye-you-cant-cal-Ra3mqb7/ (accessed 25 February 2020).

Heater, B M (2017) *30 Steps to Conscious Living*. Bloomington, IN: Balboa Press.

Jackson, K (2017) The Mindful Social Worker: How Mindfulness Can Help Social Workers Practice More Creatively. *Social Work Today*, 17(5): 14.

James, M B (2010) *The Foundation of Huna: Ancient Wisdom for Modern Times*. Hailua-Kona, HI: CreateSpace Independent Publishing Platform.

Kabat-Zinn, J (2013) *Full Catastrophe Living: Using the Wisdom of Your Body and Mind to Face Stress, Pain, and Illness*. New York: Bantam Dell.

Kahneman, D (2011) *Thinking, Fast and Slow*. London: Penguin.

Keane, W A (1994) *The Family Circus* cartoon, 31 August.

LoudLizard (nd) Negative Triangle Diagram. Courtesy of LoudLizard – Own work, CC BY-SA 3.0. [online] Available at: https://commons.wikimedia.org/w/index.php?curid=47413890 (accessed 13 February 2020).

Malinowski, P and Lim, H J (2015) Mindfulness at Work: Positive Affect, Hope, and Optimism Mediate the Relationship between Dispositional Mindfulness, Work Engagement and Well-being. [online] Available at: https://core.ac.uk/download/pdf/42476779.pdf (accessed 4 February 2020).

McGee, G Z (nd) 7 Empowering Jiddu Krishnamurti Lessons to Live By. [online] Available at: https:// fractalenlightenment.com/47675/wisdom/7-empowering-jiddu-krishnamurti-lessons-to-live-by (accessed 25 February 2020).

McLeod, S (2019) Cognitive Behavioural Therapy. [online] Available at: www.simplypsychology.org/cognitive-therapy.html (accessed 4 February 2020).

Oldale, R J (2018) Buddha, the Elephant, and the Monkey. [online] Available at: https://mastermindcontent.co.uk/buddha-the-elephant-and-the-monkey/ (accessed 4 February 2020).

Oliver, D (2002) *Polynesia in Early Historic Times*. Honolulu, HI: Bess Press.

Parker, T (2012) *Thoughts I Met on the Highway: Create the Life You Want*. Charlottesville, VA: Hampton Roads.

Rhys Davids, T W (trans) (1881) *Buddhist Suttas*. Clarendon Press.

Roeser, R W, Schonert-Reichl, K A, Jha, A, Cullen, M, Wallace, L, Wilensky, R and Harrison, J (2013) Mindfulness Training and Reductions in Teacher Stress and Burnout: Results from Two Randomized, Waitlist-control Field Trials. [online] Available at: https://miami.pure.elsevier.com/en/publications/mindfulness-training-and-reductions-in-teacher-stress-and-burnout (accessed 4 February 2020).

Rothschild, B (with Rand, M L) (2006) *Help for the Helper: The Psychophysiology of Compassion Fatigue and Vicarious Trauma*. London: W W Norton & Company.

Rutter, L and Brown, K (2012) *Critical Thinking and Professional Judgement for Social Work* (3rd ed). Post-qualifying Social Work Practice Series. London: Sage Learning Matters.

Shapiro, E (2013) Maya Angelou: 'Forgiveness Is the Greatest Gift You Can Give Yourself'. *ABC News Radio Online*. [online] Available at: http://abcnewsradioonline.com/national-news/maya-angelou-forgiveness-is-the-greatest-gift-you-can-give-y.html (accessed 25 February 2020).

Siegal, D (2010) *The Mindful Therapist: A Clinician's Guide to Mindsight and Neural Integration*. London: W W Norton & Co Ltd.

Steiner, R (1994) *Theosophy*. Hudson: Anthroposophic Press. [online] Available at: https://steiner.presswarehouse.com/sites/steiner/research/archive/theosophy/theosophy.pdf (accessed 4 February 2020).

Sturdy, C (2016) *The Twelve Attunements*. [online] Available at: www.cassandrasturdy.com/the-twelve-attunements (accessed 4 February 2020).

Taylor, B (2017) *Decision Making, Assessment and Risk in Social Work* (3rd ed). Post-qualifying Social Work Practice Series. London: Sage Learning Matters.

Tolle, E (2016) *The Power of Now*. London: Yellow Kite Publishers.

Vetter, T (1988) *The Ideas and Meditative Practices of Early Buddhism*. Leiden: Brill.

Woolfe, S (2016) *Carl Jung and Hermann Hesse Explain Why Other People Irritate Us*. 3 November. [online] Available at: https://www.samwoolfe.com/2016/11/carl-jung-and-hermann-hesse-explain-why.html (accessed 25 February 2020).

Yungen, R (2006) *A Time of Departing* (2nd ed). Eureka, MT: Lighthouse Trails Publishing.

Achieving professional emotional regulation: the impact of organisation and person

Steph

INTRODUCTION

The emotional challenges of social work practice are significant, so it can be hard to stay emotionally regulated. It's a profession where long hours combined, for many, with parental and caring responsibilities can take an inevitable emotional toll. We can be exposed to levels of trauma you could never have imagined, thus challenging the security of our attachments and our core beliefs. I know I can relate to the challenges of balancing day-to-day practice and my personal life, yet also feel, despite this, there are significant opportunities for growth and self-awareness in these challenges. I will be exploring attachment and trauma in more depth a little later in the chapter.

Emotions are a strong and powerful force and sometimes they get the better of us. They can lead us to lose focus and control, and respond in ways which, in hindsight, we wish we hadn't. Evolutionists would argue that our emotions, and the quick responses they can give us, have proved useful throughout our history. When approached by a woolly mammoth our cave dwelling ancestors got scared and ran away. That's a good reaction! Howe (2008) considers that despite our emotional reactions lacking subtlety, they are quick and powerful, placing at our disposal a range of possible immediate responses to situations we find ourselves in. Some are useful and some are less so; sometimes a better response could have been a more effectively thought through one. He suggests they are tried and tested solutions, developed over time, to the problems we all face. Emotions can make us focus on a task at hand until it is dealt with, at which point, ideally, the emotions will subside.

At the core of our emotions is a readiness to act and to formulate plans. They give a sense of urgency. The emotions you feel will 'flavour' your responses and it is useful to be able to manage these emotions in some way so that you can use your emotional responses to drive you positively rather than letting them have a negative impact. This can be hard when you have someone sitting in front of you telling you a harrowing story. You have to be able to know your emotions, know what triggers strong feelings in you, and plan for how to deal with them, rather than leaving your reactions to chance. The reality is, sometimes we don't know how we will react until we are confronted with something. We are 'forged in the fire' of practice, so to speak. Such learning requires us to be reflective practitioners.

If you haven't already, you can read more about my practice in my biography at the beginning of the book ('Steph's story' in the Introduction). But when I think about it, I can't believe I am in my twenty-third year as a social worker – that's nearly half my life in practice. I still enjoy my work and enjoy helping others increase and maintain their capacity to regulate and manage their emotions.

In my view, self-care and professional practice are distinctly linked, so my aim for this chapter is to try to give you ideas and strategies to improve both. In turn, this should help reduce the self-doubt that is often inherent in caring professionals – those awful feelings of *'am I enough?'* It is useful to understand that this is what the families, parents and service users we work with are often feeling. The first steps to understanding emotional regulation require us to draw upon neuroscience and biopsychosocial models in relation to emotional health, and consider how self-care can increase resilience; I intend to touch on these as we go along. Firstly, it is important to consider the environment in which social work takes place, as this can have an emotional impact.

THE IMPACT OF AUSTERITY ON THE SOCIAL WORK TASK

Social care and social work are always in a state of flux, and contemporary social work practice sits within times of significant practical and financial difficulties that severely challenge our practice and autonomy. Public sector cuts, reduced resources, limited services and budgets, all of which increase work-related pressures, simply place greater demands on social workers, who are expected to work harder and for longer hours. It is little wonder all this additional pressure leads to increased physical and emotional stress. Now more than ever, there is the need for us to develop genuine self-care routines to increase longevity of practice as well as our overall productivity.

While we can recognise pay freezes, cuts to car allowances and depleted training and personal development opportunities as being the result of austerity, I would say self-care has also been a casualty. As the complexity of social work has increased with reduced resources, the risk of burnout has increased (Hunter, cited in Donovan and Rushton, 2018). Furthermore, I agree with social work academic Ray Jones, who states, *'Broadly, social work is being eaten alive by austerity. The last decade saw cuts of 40 percent to council budgets, alongside increases of 70 percent in the number of child protection investigations, child protection plans and care applications'* (Jones, 2018).

In 2018, a study conducted by Bath Spa University (Ravalier and Boichat, 2018), in association with members of the Social Workers Union (SWU) and British Association for Social Work (BASW), focused upon stress and job satisfaction. Forty per cent of those interviewed indicated they wanted to leave the profession within the year. The term 'presenteeism' was described within the study to highlight workers who worked through illness at least twice a year. Children and adult services staff reported difficult work conditions, with 69 per cent of children and family social workers and 67 per cent of social workers working in adult services working through illness as they felt unable to take time off. These findings are quite worrying and highlight the need for self-care, especially within this increasingly stressful social work climate. I know that without self-care I can struggle with sleep, leading to exhaustion. This cycle can and at times does have a negative impact upon my productivity.

PERFORMANCE INDICATOR DRIVERS

Despite the 'backdrop' of austerity, I'm sure you know well enough how mandatory social work services are still driven by performance indicators to meet the Commissioner's targets. I refer to my work within Children's Mental Health Services (CAMHS), where Davies (2018) captures so well how extensive inhouse strategies have needed to be deployed to try to manage the increasing demand on services, despite services being drastically reduced. These changes are often beyond our control, yet they leaves *us* trying to manage excessive, complex workloads that require creative approaches in the face of reduced autonomy.

When the cuts emerged post-austerity, I realised the specialist mental health service I managed was likely to lose all funding, similar to many other provisions around the country. I realised I was on the losing side and sought a secondment elsewhere. I am not certain this was a 'flight' response but rather measured self-preservation, especially upon returning from maternity leave to learn of my team's relocation to 'hot-desking' in a former store cupboard! When faced with such a difficult climate to work within, our self-care is needed more than ever, but often comes last; hot-desking in particular has been associated with low morale and burnout, according to Biggart et al (2016).

In challenging times, the public sector redesigns and reconfigures. Estates management, in response to cuts, inevitably have the challenging task of trying to house staff in smaller, cheaper accommodation. I advocate being part of this and trying to embrace the changes; to quote Jean De La Fontaine, '*Je plie, et ne romps pas – I bend but do not break.*'

Embracing the changes can help us feel involved in the changes we have no control over, and that way it can feel less like '*something done to us*'. This approach to change means we develop more productive relationships with management, which can lead to greater transparency and mutual understanding of each other's needs and expectations. Trying to have input into the local implementation of national policies can help us feel like *we* have more autonomy, which can make us feel more empowered and happier in our work, meaning we in turn become much more productive.

Despite the challenges faced, I think one of my greatest achievements was delivering art groups within the NHS, which were awarded a regional NHS award for their involvement in patient recovery. Research by Kaimal et al (2016) found just 45 minutes of creative practice such as art can reduce the stress hormone cortisol. Yet, realistically, how can we measure this type of client outcome with target-driven performance indicators?

To help you I have summarised some of my self-care advice in relation to performance management as follows.

- Take an active approach to understanding the basis of national policy relating to your particular job role. For example, the move to regionalised adoption agencies is intended to share good practice and standardise services. Reading up on policy context and trying to autonomously develop specialisms or good practice to meet national, or local, standards and directives in your specialist area can help you understand and even embrace the changes. Remember change is not always a bad thing.
- Be aware of timescales for assessments and adhere to them as far as possible. Manage your diary to enable this (there's more on this in the productivity chapter, Chapter 7). Filing court reports late just stresses out other agencies, courts, families and, most of all, you!
- Work smarter, not harder! So, try to engage with partner agencies; getting to know other professionals by way of sharing resources and training (if possible) can help reduce inappropriate referrals. This in turn helps cut down some of *your* workload, meaning less stress and greater productivity.
- Endeavour to integrate self-care at work. Something as uncomplicated as a short walk at lunchtime reduces stress levels (more on this in the exercise chapter, Chapter 4).
- It is hard to ask for help as a fairly autonomous social worker, so try to find a trusted challenger, someone who can look out for you and remind you to ask for help if you are struggling (Cairns, 2002). Sometimes, all we need is someone to recognise we are having a tough time and give us a hug!
- As Confucius is believed to have said, '*When you find a job that you enjoy, you will never have to work a day in your life*'. So, focus on whatever areas of your work you really enjoy. Personally, I like the advocacy aspect and planning care with families, but since a social worker's role can be so varied choose what you like and get involved with how this service area can be delivered. Sometimes it is front-line staff who have the best ideas for how policy changes can actually work in practice!
- Use your supervision and appraisal as opportunities to discuss any areas of particular professional interest. I usually ask my staff '*What do you need to help you do your job well?*'
- Spend some time thinking about what you want to do, what you need to enable you to do this and what management support is required.

TECHNOLOGY IN SOCIAL WORK AND HARNESSING SOCIAL MEDIA

Agile working, which most of us are engaged in these days, brings with it the need to be provided with laptops and mobile phones, our work tools that allow for hot-desking. The National Association of Social Workers developed ethical standards for technology use in 2017 (NASW, 2017) but, I argue, did not consider the impact on 'us' as professionals. Social work often gets 'negative press' in the arena of social media, with affordable fingertip technology meaning that when things go wrong, everyone gets to know about it. It becomes big news, fast. What people forget is we are human. Agile working means it is probably more difficult to process upsetting information, with no guarantee of compassionate support from remote colleagues as a consequence of that distance. Scott (2019) discusses the impact of increased communication by social media, which is that while we are closer to those on the other side of the world, we are actually becoming more disconnected than connected. While agile working does have its benefits, such as flexible working, which is great if you have family commitments (this is explored in Chapter 9), many colleagues have told me they have developed poor coping mechanisms such as constantly checking and responding to work-related emails while on annual leave. This means they never really truly disconnect from work when not at work. Personally, I have found significant value in professional support, peer supervision and access to like-minded colleagues to aid debriefing, especially when dealing with challenging situations. I think this is an area where organisations need to give some more serious consideration to methods of reducing the potential isolation of social workers in a digital age, especially as it appears it is here to stay.

THE VALUE OF NEUROSCIENCE

Just as digital gadgets are always being improved and developed, neuroscience is one of the areas of greatest scientific development in the last decade. We now know more about the impact of trauma and toxic stress on the brain, and on physical and mental health, than we did ten years ago. Not looking after oneself can have important neurological consequences.

I tend to give a really simple explanation regarding neuroscience and biology to help families and professionals.

I will use the example of teenagers. Adolescence is one of the most developmentally sensitive periods in life. Physical changes are constant. In the UK, the onset of puberty is getting earlier, sometimes occurring during primary school years, which has been linked to increased consumption of processed food and to childhood obesity. Children's bodies developing before their brains can be linked to a higher risk of mental health problems.

Adolescence is not just a period in which teenagers form their identity but is also a period of brain growth and a time when greater amounts of sleep are required. If trauma occurs during adolescence (for example, if a young person being bullied, which can expose them to prolonged fear), cortisol levels increase and in turn there is a reduction in dopamine transmitters, leading to lower mood and poor concentration. This may also impact on the pituitary gland's production of melatonin, thus diminishing sleep which is critical for healthy development during adolescence.

Hold this example in mind while you consider neuroscience and the impact of stress at work when we revisit this a little later.

THE CRUCIAL IMPORTANCE OF THERAPEUTIC AND REFLECTIVE WORKSPACE

Now, of course this is a self-care book about *you* and looking after *yourself* as a practitioner. The example above is about adolescence, but I have included it because I find that as social workers we do struggle to place our needs first. We are much better at considering ideas for others than following our own advice! I find understanding the neuroscience and biological impact of trauma on service users can actually help social workers to think about the impact that hearing about trauma can have on them. This is termed 'secondary trauma'.

I have learned over the years that social workers tend not to think of themselves or consider how to improve their emotional regulation. Medical friends of mine tell me they would never allow their weekly continuing professional development (CPD) time to be absorbed into clinical work. Yet, social workers struggle to impose these personal boundaries on things such as training and supervision. How many times have you cancelled training because you have a court report that has to be completed and submitted?

If we look towards therapeutic space to aid children and young people's biological, emotional and social needs as being important, recreating a supportive work environment that considers these things can be just as vital. With gentle encouragement and the provision of therapeutic thinking space, I believe, social workers can discuss the impact of cases on their biological, psychological and social selves in a safe and confidential environment, thus utilising a biopsychosocial model to consider their own needs.

Earlier there was a simple illustration of what can be happening biologically and emotionally with adolescence. Now let's apply it to self-care.

Mary is a middle-aged social worker and single mum. Slim all her life, the last few years she has found this harder to maintain. She wonders if this is linked to the stress hormone, which is known to lead to increased weight gain, especially around the tummy area. Mary is tired due to her workload; she can work late into the evening on the laptop as she cannot find time for some things in her working day. Mary is not sleeping well and is often overeating when tired or making less healthy food choices. She can catastrophise things and thinks if she does not do certain tasks, her employment will be affected. Mary takes social work values seriously; she thinks she could let down families she supports and often feels overstretched.

It is understood cortisol can also suppress the immune system, as can alcohol and tobacco. McEwen (2013) explains that sleep deprivation creates significant difficulties including elevated evening cortisol, insulin and blood pressure, as well as elevated gut hormones increasing appetite. Long-term sleep deprivation can lead to weight gain, depression and cognitive impairment. He emphasises that the brain is key in determining how we respond to stress. Past experiences of bullying, abuse and trauma, including secondary trauma, will increase hypervigilance and the brain may be more hardwired in flight or fight responses.

Protective factors including supportive adults, an easy temperament and problem-solving skills may increase individual resilience and capacity to manage stress. McEwen's (2013) research indicates that chronic stress over 21 days impairs hippocampus-dependent cognitive functioning and increases fear conditioning responses which impact negatively on emotional regulation.

Clearly there are strong biological and neuroscience arguments for increasing self-care to manage stress and increase productivity. What could Mary do in terms of her own self-care?

COMPASSION FOCUSED THERAPY

Compassion is a human behavioural quality that is evident when we support others and show warmth and empathy. It can increase dopamine and reduce cortisol levels as it increases responses in the reward part of the brain leading to joy and altruism. Put simply, we regulate our emotions better when we connect with others; it helps us feel better about our own issues and concerns when we help others with theirs.

> *It is our lack of love for ourselves that inhibits our compassion towards others. If we make friends with ourselves, then there is no obstacle to opening our hearts and minds to others.*
>
> (The Happy Buddha, 2015, p 9)

Compassion focused therapy (CFT) is designed to encourage compassion towards self and others. It is derived from Buddhist or humanistic approaches. This type of approach, in my view, is particularly useful for social workers, who can be notoriously self-critical. It is drawn from psychotherapy and helps you step back and consider why you may be thinking in a certain way.

For example, a tool I use is called 'compassionate friend'. If in supervision a social worker or social work student says, '*I am rubbish, I cannot keep up with the workload, I am not cut out for this work*', I will ask them, '*If you were the friend or social work colleague of the person saying that, what would you say to them? Would you allow them to be so self-critical?*'

I would then ask them to explore professional, environmental and even societal challenges which impact upon their work and help them separate these factors from the personal aspects. I usually find in taking this approach people can see that they are less kind and more self-critical to themselves than they would ever be to others. When their negative inner voices are spoken aloud, people usually then accept how unhelpful they are. Given social workers agree to work by professional values, and compassion is a core value, it is vital we learn to be compassionate to ourselves. CFT is a tool that works as effectively with ourselves as it does with service users. Lisa talks more about compassion and self-forgiveness within her chapter on mindfulness and spirituality (Chapter 5).

POWER TOGETHER AND CO-PRODUCTION

We know that for many, to improve their lives or situations often requires a change. This applies to us just as much as it does to the service users we work with. 'Power Together' models and models of co-production allow reciprocity and harnessing an individual's assets and strengths, according to Dix et al (2019), resulting in more positive outcomes.

We have explained elsewhere in various places (see especially Chapter 3) how during our fight or flight response cortisol levels increase, which aids our ability to respond to danger. However, long-term exposure to stress or secondary trauma can dull our fight or flight responses. What that means is people become used to their daily stress, they normalise it and become immune to the stress they are experiencing and don't see the need to change.

Let's think about this for a moment. If a bear came into my garden, I'm certain I would want to run! But if the bear came into my garden every day, I would get used to seeing the bear and become less fearful of it. Taking a fight or flight approach, on the bear's first visit my stress response would be activated, yet exposure to this fear by seeing a bear each day would inevitably dull my response. Like a leaky tap, the slow drip, drip, drip exposure to this stress normalises it.

So, when we work with families who have undergone a period of chronic stress and trauma, we can observe they can lose their capacity to regulate emotions. We too, as social workers, are at risk of the same thing as a consequence of the work we do. Repeated exposure to observing the trauma of our clients causes our cortisol levels to increase and we risk burnout or secondary trauma as we become immune to its impact. Cairns (2002) describes trauma as 'catching' as a consequence of engaging in toxic stress. She advocates the importance of working in a team to reduce the risk of second-ary trauma emerging. The team's compassion and reflective space will provide a buffer and increase resilience. While agile working often makes this more difficult, this therefore emphasises the importance for us all to develop *and practise* self-care, such as exercise, gardening, art and meditation, so that the risk of long-term damage as a result of irregular cortisol levels can be reduced or avoided.

BIOPSYCHOSOCIAL MODEL OF TRAUMA

I always find it helpful to consider Engel's biopsychosocial model of trauma, first intro-duced in the 1960s (Adler, 2009), in relation to my work and private life. I know that when I am under periods of intense stress biologically I can end up with headaches and an upset stomach. The social impact is I might socialise less, which has a negative impact on my general well-being, especially as I am a social person and socialising helps me unwind and manage my stress. So, for me, staying home because I am not physically well is not a useful strategy.

THE IMPACT OF BIOPSYCHOSOCIAL INJURY

It is important to get to know yourself and how you respond to stress. I know staying home is not a useful stress buster for me. I do know the importance of developing effective self-care strategies, including learning to listen to the signals my body sends me when stressed. As soon as I can feel a headache start, I know that is my body telling me it's time to slow down. The following are examples of how stress can affect us, and I'm confident you will recognise some of them:

- headaches;
- flashbacks;
- withdrawal from social activities;

- tummy upsets;
- hypervigilance;
- performance anxiety;
- vocal and facial tics;
- scanning for threats;
- social anxiety;
- tremors;
- guilt and shame;
- isolation.

APPLYING THEORY TO PRACTICE TO STRENGTHEN SKILLS AND PRODUCTIVITY

How many times as a social work student did you hear said or say yourself, '*You need to apply theory to practice*'? Knowing underpinning theories and legislation makes us feel more skilled and confident in our professional role, helping us to perform well, and it's the same for self-care. We need to take that knowledge and put it into practice. If we put into practice even the smallest self-care steps, we can expand our capacity to work more efficiently and be more productive in the workplace. If we feel like we can manage our workload, we feel more confident and happier. A study by Oswald et al (2015), economists at the University of Warwick, found that happiness leads to a 12 per cent increase in productivity. Interestingly the same study found that workers who are unhappy are 10 per cent less productive than their happier colleagues.

In today's world of social work, the work we do can be so challenging that we end up developing dysfunctional coping mechanisms. For example, the nutrition chapter (Chapter 3), 'Rubbish in, rubbish out', highlights the difference between good intentions and practice reality. We are all trying our best at self-care and when we manage it well with honest reflection on our practice this reflection increases productivity. Engel, who I mentioned earlier, is a psychiatrist who developed the biopsychosocial model and applied it to health. He pioneered thinking in relation to the intrinsic links between emotional and physical health (Engel, 1977).

I use this model to underpin my practice, particularly in relation to trauma. I believe this model helps us 'listen' to ourselves more. When teaching, I ask professionals to consider their well-being and how they can achieve optimum emotional and biological health. I ask them to link emotional states and well-being by mapping out any symptoms they are currently experiencing and connecting them to areas of difficulties they may be facing in work or life in general. This is also a really useful tool to use within the safe confines of supervision, as it can help you, as a worker, to identify your symptoms and make plans to manage these. See the box below for an idea of how this works in practice.

Start with a piece of paper and make three columns:

- biological;
- psychological;
- social and environmental.

Think about each of these areas in turn and consider difficulties you are having in each area. For example, the biological column might have something like '*can't get to sleep*'. The psychological column may have '*I'm worrying about a case at work*'. And the social and environmental column may include '*I've prioritised bringing my laptop home to do some work over going to an exercise class I like*'.

Take the time to think about the self-care strategies (if any) you currently use, which can be either positive or negative. How do they help you overcome the above difficulties?

Do your self-care strategies make things worse, eg the impact of drinking a bottle of wine?

Think about what you could do differently. Then, go to the relevant chapter in the book and see what and how you could do things differently!

PSYCHODYNAMIC THEORIES

Psychodynamic theories originate from Freud (1930). He felt the unconscious has a powerful impact on our behaviour. He proposed that childhood experiences impact significantly on adulthood behaviour, thought processes and relationships. Rohner (2016) built on this by researching the impact rejection can have on the brain. His study discovered the pain centre of the brain was activated in those research participants who had first-hand experience of rejection. If you work within the field of substance misuse, you will no doubt be familiar with this concept, given the number of abuse survivors who self-medicate with substances just to cope with day-to-day life. Knowing and understanding the outcome of this type of research helps us to provide psychoeducation to survivors of abuse. It is invaluable to be able to explain how there is a clinical physiological reason for their behaviour, as this can really liberate survivors from the shame and guilt that may increase with their misuse of substances.

Likewise, it is vital we know and understand how, when working with clients, transference can happen. I think of this as me being handed a 'parcel of guilt'. The guilt and shame felt by service users can be passed to us as the social worker. Imagine a client saying to you '*Here take this parcel of guilt. You fix these problems.*' People often see us as being the ones who have all the answers to their problems and they can get upset when we don't. What is not always considered is that, alongside our professional demands, we also need to manage these emotional demands.

EMOTIONAL REGULATION

Emotions are funny things; they can be triggered and bubble up from almost nowhere. When exploring emotions, a good starting point is to develop an understanding of what I refer to as 'emotional regulation'. I first came across this term during 'Theraplay' training. Theraplay is a therapeutic approach developed by Booth and Jernberg (2009). It's a model that focuses on the application of attachment theory to clinical practice, in order to improve attachment relationships, and a child's ability to regulate big and strong adult-like feelings.

Most of the families we work with experience significant emotional dysregulation. Many are unable to cope with powerful feelings such as envy, rage and despair, and they don't always have the necessary coping skills or understanding to manage them. That is why psychoeducation is crucial in mental health social work. It is an evidence-based intervention involving practical information for families to enable them to understand the difficulties they are experiencing.

Let's consider this in practice with a case example and then think about issues for you as a social worker:

Bethany, aged 13, lives with her grandmother, Betty. Bethany has a diagnosis of attention deficit hyperactivity disorder (ADHD). Betty has special guardianship in respect of Bethany, as Bethany's mother, Clare, misuses heroin. Clare struggled with substances after experiencing sexual abuse as a child, perpetrated by Betty's uncle. Bethany wants to have a close relationship with her mother, Clare, but this has proved difficult as she has found Clare to be unreliable over the years.

Betty, the grandmother, becomes very angry with Mary, their social worker. Betty can swear at Mary and threaten to place Bethany in care. These threats have Mary feeling so stressed that she can feel her chest tighten when she needs to phone Betty.

Mary thinks she is failing Bethany but is also angry, as she feels Betty probably contributed to Clare's heroin problems.

Think about what Mary could do to regulate her emotions better when feeling stressed before she phones Betty. What would she want to consider when thinking about Betty's attitude towards her?

How could Mary improve her response in terms of her self-care?

DEVELOPING EMOTIONAL INTELLIGENCE

If we take a moment to reflect upon the above case study, we can see how explosive emotions can be, especially the ones Mary is experiencing as within that situation she needs to remain objective and professional. Recognising and managing your emotions as well as managing the emotions of others is known as emotional intelligence. Goleman (1996) suggests that there are three emotional 'styles' that people exhibit.

Some people are 'engulfed'. They can feel swamped by their emotions and helpless to control them. Their mood takes charge and they get lost or overwhelmed by their emotional response to things. They can lack perspective, the ability to stand back and analyse what is really going on.

Others are 'accepting'. They are clear about how they are feeling and accept the moods that they experience. Crucially, though, they do nothing to change the emotions they are feeling, rather they just ride that emotional wave, not particularly overwhelmed nor seeking to do anything about it.

Finally, some people are 'self-aware'. They are aware of their mood and have what Goleman (1996) refers to as a sophisticated response to it. They are clear about their emotions, are sure about their boundaries and, most crucially, they are mindful (see Chapter 5 for more on mindfulness).

I wonder, which one are you? Take a moment to ponder!

Goleman (1996) suggests there are five domains to consider regarding emotional intelligence. First, you need to know your emotions. You need to develop the ability to identify your feelings as they happen, through close monitoring of self, as if you don't, then you are at the mercy of them. Second, you need to know how to manage your emotions. This relies on developing strategies from self-awareness. Goleman notes that having poor skills in this area leads to distress, while those with good skills have the ability to 'bounce back' during difficult times. Third, he goes on to state that motivating yourself is crucial. Mastering your emotions assists in areas that enhance productivity, such as being able to pay attention, being creative and getting into the 'flow'. Controlling your emotions restricts impulsiveness and helps you think critically. Next, he suggests being emotionally intelligent helps recognise the emotions in others. This helps develop empathy and helps you attune to the subtle signals that people give, often without even realising. Finally, he states that emotional intelligence is key to handling relationships. Surely this is what social work is all about!

As we develop our emotional intelligence, we need to keep it constantly under review. It is not a static quality and it will be challenged both by the service users we work with, who are often in emotional turmoil themselves, and by the demands placed on us by the organisations we work in.

The role of reflection – either on your own, with others, or formally in supervision – is crucial. Reflection 'in action' helps us to explore what is happening as it is happening. Reflection 'on action', on the other hand, helps us analyse and think critically about what has happened and what we could have done differently. For example, how could Mary have approached her discussions with Betty differently to reduce the likelihood of Betty becoming angry?

Edwards (2017) advocates moving beyond this traditional 'in action' and 'on action' approach, suggesting another two areas. She puts forward the idea that we should start with reflection 'before' action. This helps us to build emotional resilience by identifying beforehand potential triggers for our emotions and in turn allows us to devise possible solutions should such emotions arise. For example, if Mary had reflected upon her feelings of anger towards Betty for her treatment of Clare before speaking to her, she might have handled her telephone discussion with Betty, and thus managed Betty's anger towards her, more effectively. Was her approach clouded by her views?

Edwards goes on to explain how reflecting 'beyond' action helps move the practitioner beyond a simple narrative. It facilitates ongoing building of professional resilience as well as promoting confidence and self-mastery, which we have seen elsewhere (eg Chapter 1) helps us develop 'flow' in our work. It builds knowledge and skills and looks for development needs through a *'What could I have done differently?'* approach.

CONCLUSION

There is no moving away from the fact that reflection is key to all we do as social workers, for the reason that we are not born with an innate ability to self-regulate. Instead, we develop this as we move from childhood into adulthood and often learn by co-regulating with others. Social work is a team activity and I cannot stress enough the importance of considering the three areas described in the biopsychosocial model when we think about self-care and how the different elements interact. Even though our working lives are more digital than ever, we still need our colleagues and managers for support with good quality, compassionate supervision. The lasting message I hope you have gained from this chapter is to be kind to yourselves. Be compassionate with yourself. Be thoughtful about the care you give yourself while you are working diligently to help others. You, like them, are important.

FURTHER READING

Blades, R, Ronicle, J, Selwyn, J and Ottaway, H (2018) *Evaluation of Regional Adoption Agencies: Inception and Scoping Report*. November 2018. Bristol: Bristol University.

Cohen, S (1972) *Folk Devils and Moral Panics: The Creation of Mods and Rockers*. London: Routledge.

Dyke, C (2019) *Writing Analytical Assessments in Social Work*. St Albans: Critical Publishing.

Hammond, N (2019) ADHD: The role of Dopamine. *Psychiatric Genetics*, 25(3): 119–26.

Kahneman, D (2011) *Thinking, Fast and Slow*. London: Penguin.

Mental Health Foundation (2009) *In the Face of Fear: How Fear and Anxiety Affect Our Health and Society, and What We Can Do About It*. London: Mental Health Foundation.

Moran, H (2015) The Coventry Grid. Differences between Autistic Spectrum Disorder (ASD) and Attachment Problems Based upon Clinical Experiences and Observations. [online] Available at: www2.oxfordshire.gov.uk/cms/sites/default/files/folders/documents/virtualschool/processesandforms/resourcesandpublications/CoventryGrid.pdf (accessed 25 February 2020).

Parton, N and Williams, S (2017) The Contemporary Refocusing of Children's Services in England. *Journal of Children's Services*, 12(2/3): 85–96.

Shoesmith, S (2017) *Learning from Baby Peter: The Politics of Blame, Fear and Denial*. London: Jessica Kingsley Publishers.

Tew, J (2006) Understanding Power and Powerlessness: Towards a Framework for Emancipatory Practice in Social Work. *Journal of Social Work*, 6(1): 33–51.

White, M (2007) *Maps of Narrative Practice*. New York: Norton Professional Books.

REFERENCES

Adler, R H (2009) Engel's Biopsychosocial Model Is Still Relevant Today. *Journal of Psychosomatic Research* 67(6): 607–11.

Biggart, L, Ward, E, Cook, L, Stride, C, Schofield, G, Corr, P, Fletcher, C, Bowler, J, Jordan, P and Bailey, S (2016) Emotional Intelligence and Burnout in Child and Family Social Work: Implications for Policy and Practice. Centre for Research on Children and Families, University of East Anglia. [online] Available at: https://www.uea.ac.uk/documents/5802799/13173245/UEA+EI+SWK+Research+Briefing+June+2016+F INAL.pdf/196909c2-69fe-44bc-9ee7-cafa62eafac4 (accessed 25 February 2020).

Booth, P B and Jernberg, A M (2009) *Theraplay*. San Francisco, CA: Jossey-Bass.

Cairns, K (2002) *Attachment, Trauma and Resilience: Therapeutic Caring for Children*. London: BAAF.

Davies, C (2018) Mental Health Services for the Young Is NHS Silent Catastrophe. *The Guardian*, 24 June 2018.

Dix, H, Hollinrake, S and Meade, J (2019) *Relationship-based Social Work with Adults*. St Albans: Critical Publishing.

Donovan, C and Rushton, P (2018) *Austerity: A Bad Idea in Practice*. London: Palgrave Macmillan.

Edwards, S (2017) Reflecting Differently. New Dimensions: Reflection-before-action and Reflection-beyond-action. *International Practice Journal*, 7(1): 1–14. doi:10.19043/ipdj.71.002.

Engel, G (1977) The Need for a New Medical Model: A Challenge for Biomedical Science. *Science*, 196: 126–9.

Freud, S (1930) *A General Introduction to Psychoanalysis*. London: Wordsworth Press.

Goleman, D (1996) *Emotional Intelligence. Why It Can Matter More Than IQ*. London: Bloomsbury Publishing.

Howe, D (2008) *The Emotionally Intelligent Social Worker*. Basingstoke: Palgrave Macmillan.

Jones (2018) *In Whose Interest? The Privatisation of Child Protection and Social Work*. Bristol: Press.

Kaimal, G, Kendra, R and Muniz, J (2016) Reduction of Cortisol Levels and Participants' Responses Following Art-making. *Art Therapy Journal of American Art Therapy Association*, 33(7): 74–80.

McEwen, B S (2013) The Brain on Stress: Towards an Integrative Approach to Brain, Body and Behaviour. *Perspective of Psychological Science*, 8(6): 673–5.

NASW (National Association of Social Workers) (2017) *Code of Ethics*. Washington, DC: NASW.

Oswald, A J, Proto, E and Sgroi, D (2015) Happiness and Productivity. *Journal of Labor Economics*, 33(4): 789–822.

Ravalier, J M and Boichat, C (2018) UK Social Workers: Working Conditions and Wellbeing. Bath Spa University. [online] Available at: www.basw.co.uk/system/files/resources/Working%20Conditions%20%20Stress%20%282018%29%20pdf.pdf (accessed 25 February 2020).

Rohner, R P (2016) Introduction to Interpersonal Acceptance-Rejection Theory (IPARTheory) and Evidence. *Online Readings in Psychology and Culture*, 6(1). doi:10.9707/2307-0919.1055.

Scott, H (2019) Understanding Links between Social Media Use, Sleep and Mental Health. Recent Progress and Current Challenges. *Current Sleep Medicine Reports*, 5(3): 141–9.

The Happy Buddha (2015) *Mindfulness and Compassion*. Lewes: Leaping Hare Press.

7 Being organised to fuel productivity: how do you know what you need to do and how do you do it?

Stephen

INTRODUCTION: DEFINING THE PROBLEM

When I ask people how organised they are I get a range of responses. Many people are 'being organised' experts and many people simply respond with a shake of their head and follow it up with some mutterings about being very last minute and out of control. There are then a group of people who fall in between these groups and, in reality, that's probably where most of us fall. We're organised sometimes, in some ways, but at other times we exist in a world of mild chaos. I imagine you are reading this because you want to be more organised than you already are, no matter where you are at on that continuum. While as a professional practitioner you are in essence employed to work with people, you inevitably end up as a manager of information and knowledge. Lots of jobs are like that now. It is in that aspect of our work where we need to be organised so we can actually get at, and get on with, the part of the profession that attracted us to it in the first place.

What has struck me in talking to people about managing yourself and being productive in the workplace is that it is clearly a skill that not everyone naturally has. This is useful to know. Diary management, prioritising, planning ahead and thinking work tasks through is not common sense and people have varying degrees of skill in these areas. These skills are crucial in managing any workplace, and more so when the psychological demands of working at supporting people either with their education, or with their community access, or with their health conditions, are added in. We have become managers of information and systems as well as managing the needs of service users. We have to balance the competing needs of our organisation, and often other organisations, while trying to meet deadlines, be focused and 'in the moment' when with people, and make sure we are up to date with the latest legal and practice changes (Wray and Rymell, 2014). No wonder workplace stress is a significant factor to contend with.

Experiencing stress in our day-to-day work usually transforms itself into big statements like, '*I'm going to have a paperwork day*', '*I'm going to make a to do list*', '*I'm going to start again on Monday and get myself sorted*', with these thoughts generally resulting in putting the kettle on and making a round of coffees for colleagues. We all seem to be experts at putting things off!

So why don't we simply give up hope and just continue trying to muddle through? Well, that's simple. It's not good for our mental health to feel on the back foot all of the time, to be constantly wondering what we should do next or what we might have forgotten to do. These things eat away at what psychologists call our psychological capital. Without psychological capital we will not have the space in our heads to be 'in the moment' with people, or to remain focused on a task until completion. Does that feel familiar? What we need is a system supported by some productivity techniques that manages all of the routine for us, leaving us to engage in professional person-focused practice.

The problem in the modern professional workplace is the volume of information we are asked to manage. It is said we can only manage to hold about seven items in our short-term working memory at any one time. With more than that number of things to work with we risk forgetting things or we become quickly overwhelmed trying to contemplate all of the tasks we have to do. Allen (2015) refers to these as 'open loops'. Open loops go around and round in our working memory while we try to both work on tasks and remember our open loops. Open loops drain our capacity to be productive. Allen suggests that we need to externalise these open loops. He observes something which we all instinctively know which is that memory is not a reliable thing. If memory was a reliable thing you wouldn't still have light bulbs needing to be changed or torches without batteries even though you've been to the supermarket many times and reminded yourself of what you needed before you went!

Heylighen and Vidal (2007) note that our long-term memory is good at noting patterns and appropriate actions but poor at recall. You will have experienced this when trying to recall someone's name. You recognise the person in front of you but can't quite place them when out of context. We need that contextualised information to support our recall. Once things are recalled and we have them in our working memory we struggle to keep them there while engaging in thinking because the two elements, remembering and thinking, interfere with each other and quickly lead to fatigue and ultimately forgetting. That's the 'Now, where was I?' phenomenon, when you have been distracted by something and then have to pick up where you left off (Heylighen and Vidal, 2007).

The 'being organised' element of our work requires the externalising of memories so that we are given triggers for action at the appropriate point in time without having to remember. The 'Getting Things Done' methodology of David Allen (2015), which I will draw on (among others) in this chapter, takes a pragmatic 'bottom up' approach to managing the work that needs to be done (asking, 'What are the tasks?') rather than a 'top down', 'what are the abstract goals?', approach. While it does start with what needs to be achieved it still works in tangible end products to achieve the bigger goal. This gives it a very concrete feel and gives actionable, practical steps to get us to where we need to be (Allen, 2015; Heylighen and Vidal, 2007).

This 'being organised' takes discipline. Finding success in this, though, according to Keller and Papasan (2014, p 55), is 'a short race'. They say this because being organised is habit forming. Once you do it and feel the benefit of it you will find you can't stop doing it – and the feeling of being in control, even when concerned by how much there is to do, is a really good one. If you can know what is to do and can select the one thing that needs to be done, then you are on the road to success. Once you form a habit it is hard to break it, as I'm sure you know from some of the negative habits you will have, like I do! Building good organising habits promotes productivity.

WHAT ARE THE PROBLEMS?

The work context

Let's accept we will never be caught up! The demands of professional life and the 'do more with less' approach that has been adopted in these times of austerity and cutbacks mean we will never be done. There will always be something to so. Just as fast as you are getting things done other things will come into your sphere of responsibility. Keeping track of these things needs to be a priority or you will constantly feel like you may have forgotten something.

Professional life does not take place in a static environment. If you worked on a production line you could largely predict how your day would pan out. This is not the case in professional practice with people. The service users we work for sometimes don't do the things we would expect, or events emerge in their lives that were unexpected, or they forget to mention crucial pieces of information. There is a requirement to be ready and able to respond on a frequent basis to urgent requests that involve rethinking our own goals and priorities for the day or even the week (Wray and Rymell, 2014). Having a trusted system you can turn to which will show you what you have to do, so that you can quickly reorganise and respond, is essential (Allen, 2015).

Overwhelm

Have you ever found yourself sitting at your desk not knowing what to do next? Disabled by the work that is in front of you? Sometimes not even sure, completely, what exactly is in front of you? You simply don't know what do next and as a consequence feel demotivated to do anything? That is overwhelm.

There are several things you can do to help overcome this state of inertia or avoid getting there in the first place. Later in this chapter we'll look at some ideas that I can assure you I use and that help.

Firstly, you need a trusted system that contains everything that is within your sphere of responsibility. It must include everything that you need to do something about. The trusted system is an 'all or nothing' system. If it doesn't contain everything then it might as well contain nothing because you will always wonder if it does, in fact, contain everything. The payoff for taking the time to develop a trusted system is that you are not storing anything in your mind so your mind will be clear to focus on the next task (Allen, 2015). There's more on creating your trusted system later in the chapter.

Secondly you need an effective way to prioritise what you have to do. You need to spend some time planning your working day. Making today good starts with what you did yesterday. It is essential to develop a planning routine. I spend time in planning mode at the start and end of each day. I then have a 'last thing Friday' planning session, and then every month I have a 'three months ahead' planning session. There's a great visual metaphor that you may have seen on social media. The professor at the front of the class takes a jar and puts big rocks into it. He asks the class if the jar is full and they say it is because no more big rocks will fit in. He then takes pebbles and pours them into the jar and the pebbles work their way in between the big rocks. He asks if the jar is full now and their reply again is yes. He then proceeds to pour sand into the jar, filling the crevices left by the rocks and pebbles. But he isn't finished there. He then pours water into the jar and eventually the jar is full. The point of this demonstration is that you need to put your rocks in first because if you start by filling the jar with pebbles you won't get the rocks in. They won't fit between the pebbles. Or if you filled it with sand first you wouldn't get the rocks or pebbles in. If you fill your 'jar' with less important, less high value things first you will have no room left when you need to put such a large thing in your 'jar', and you will become overwhelmed.

> Think about all of the things you need to get done.
> These will be things in your working life and your personal life.
> Which of these things are your 'rocks' that you need to get in there first?
> Which are your 'pebbles'?
> Is there anything you keep putting into your jar that you should stop putting in there?
> Write your answers down and put them somewhere safe.

You need to plan regularly to make sure your big rocks are in your 'trusted system' first before adding in other things. This leads to another problem, which is often referred to as the 'planning fallacy', and that is our tendency to underestimate how long big tasks take and overestimate how long small tasks take. This is because we tend to base our judgement of how long something will take on a best-case scenario, the time when we wrote that report in an hour, rather than an average of the times it can take us to write a report. The average inevitably will be longer than the best version (Webb, 2017). Planning requires a critical look at what there is to do and how long it will take. We'll explore how to do this later in the chapter.

The myth of multitasking

The productivity literature is unanimous in its view that '*multitasking is a lie*' (Keller and Papasan, 2014, p 44) but, worse, it's actually detrimental to productivity. We all intuitively know that our brains find it difficult to cope with two things at once. How many of us when driving on open road have the radio on loud and when we get to the car park and need to concentrate to park the car turn the radio down or off and say, '*I can't hear myself think!*' You can listen to the music and get lost in it when you are on 'automatic pilot' but when you need to focus on a task that requires your full attention you've got to turn the music down!

To consider why multitasking does in fact slow us down I want to give you a computer related analogy. You power your laptop up and you start work. You need to read your emails, so you run your email program. You need to open a word document from an email so your word processor launches. To respond to an email, you need some information from a spreadsheet, so you run your spreadsheet program. You decide to have some music while you work so you start to stream something online. Emails keep dropping into your inbox, music keeps playing, you keep typing into your document, you switch between your emails and your spreadsheet for information, and all is well. The laptop appears to be doing everything all at once! The reality is that all it is doing is switching between tasks. Doing a little bit of this task then a little bit of the next task and eventually, when you have too many programs running for your machine to cope with, it all becomes too much for it and you get the dreaded symbol that means *'Hang on, I'm trying to catch up'*. And then if it all gets too much… crash! And we have to reboot and start again.

If you are trying to do this in your work life, your productivity will be negatively affected. You might well think you are able to tune into the conversation your colleagues are having, while responding to an email, while making sure you remember to make that phone call to a service user, but in reality you can't. This scenario is made worse by other distractions we encounter. Your email 'buzzes' to tell you something has arrived. You phone 'pings' with a Facebook update. Your phone rings and you have to take the call. And then crash! You forget the phone call you have to make and you make errors in the report. If you are 'running' too many tasks at once something will get forgotten or not done very well.

Rene Marois at Vanderbilt University (Dux et al, 2006) showed that doing two tasks at the same time took 30 per cent longer than doing them sequentially and there were twice as many errors in the finished tasks. A study by Iqbal and Horvitz (2007) showed that after an interruption to read email it took 10 to 15 minutes to return to focused activity on the task that was originally being undertaken. As Keller and Papasan (2014, p 75) state, *'in an effort to attend to all things, everything gets short-changed and nothing gets its due'*.

The impact is also real in terms of the chemistry of your brain and therefore your well-being. Levitin (2015) tells us that multitasking creates a dopamine addiction as we engage with new stimuli, thwarting our ability to stay focused as we must go and look at the thing demanding our attention. Think about the little rush you get when something pops up on Facebook or Twitter that you must look at to see who has 'liked' your post. Our prefrontal cortex, the bit of our brain trying to keep us focused, gets drawn into the new fascinating thing and we have lost the impetus for the task in hand. Particularly problematic in terms of our well-being and self-care is that it has been found that multitasking increases *'the production of the stress hormone cortisol as well as the fight or flight hormone adrenaline which can overstimulate your brain and cause mental fog or scrambled thinking'* (Levitin, 2015, p 96). In our potentially already stressed state our multitasking actions have increased our bodies' chemical stress responses.

SOLUTIONS

So, there are some things that clearly get in the way of our productivity but what's the solution?! We'll explore this next but the words that come to mind when I think of solutions are being focused, productive, engaged in planning, structured and organised. If all is well, I'm motivated. If things are all in order, I have time to be a reflective practitioner and to focus on deep thinking and professional development. We need a whole-system, holistic, approach to the day so that we can be in the 'flow'. What we are aiming for is psychological well-being through meaningful and mindful work (Allen, 2015).

The best way to explore some of the methods you can employ is to talk you through how I stay organised and focused on a daily, weekly and monthly basis. The methods I will share with you need effort to employ them to start with but once they become ingrained in the way you work, part of the positive self-care habits you form, you won't be able to stop yourself from doing them. Let me give you an example. A student stops me after a lecture and asks me if we can meet up for a tutorial. As soon as they are talking, I sense myself psychologically going for my diary (which is electronic so is available on my smartphone). As they talk, I listen and maybe ask what they want to talk about. I'm thinking all the time '*Is this something we can deal with quickly, does it need a longer amount of time, or is it something that needs some preparation and planning?*'. Once I know this, I'm already checking my calendar. Can I do it right now? Can I give the student a time to meet later? Can I ask the student to do something to help with the planning? Depending on the answer to these questions and others, either the conversation happens straight away and it's done, and I can put it out of my head, or a task is handed back to the student by asking them to email me with some times they can meet, or it's in my diary as an action for me to pick up when I next have time. Whichever of those options it is, after the moment we are engaged in, the thing is over and it is safe to be forgotten. It's not stored in my brain. Either it's dealt with, or the student has something to do and I'll be reminded to do something when they provide me with something, or it's 'remembered' in my calendar. My psychological capacity is intact without having an 'open loop' whirring around in my brain with me trying desperately to remember what it is I need to do at some point in the future. My trusted system is doing the work for me. Let's look at some solutions.

The 'trusted system'

This phrase the 'trusted system' comes from productivity guru David Allen. His book *Getting Things Done, the Art of Stress-free Productivity* is a best-seller and I would highly recommend it. It was the starting point for me of everything in this book. Allen (2015) states that we need a trusted system that reminds us of everything we need to do when we need to do it. The trusted system is an all or nothing system. It captures everything that is in your sphere of responsibility that you may need to do now, soon, sometime and 'someday-maybe'. What you use as a 'system' is up to you. You can use anything from pen and paper to computer-based solutions. My trusted system is a combination of a spreadsheet and an electronic calendar.

It's not easy to get your system up and running and it takes some effort because you need to take everything recorded anywhere that you need to do, including all of the things stored in your mind, and get it all into your trusted system. Allen (2015) refers to this externalising of the things in your mind as a mind dump.

When I started this, I worked on it, on and off, for a couple of weeks. While working on it anything that I was asked to do went straight into the system, bypassing my other methods. First, I transferred my paper diary into my electronic calendar. I then created a spreadsheet with various tabs for each of the major activities I engage in at work: one for each module I run, one for the student placements I organise, one for student shadowing opportunities, and so on. I then got together the various piles of paper, notebooks and sticky notes I had and started to work my way through them. Anything that was date and time specific went into the calendar as a specific date and time event. Anything that felt like it needed to be done soon but wasn't time and date specific went in as an all-day event on a day where I felt I might be able to do it. Tasks or ideas that were not time and date specific or that were ideas that needed to be developed went into the appropriate tab on the spreadsheet to be considered at a later date. I then did a 'mind dump'. I sat with a notepad and wrote down everything I could think of that was stuck in my head. Thinking of one thing naturally prompted me to think of other things. Once I had all of this, I put it into the calendar or spreadsheet.

Allen (2015, p 12) says that '*Your ability to generate power* [motivation and forward direction] *is directly proportional to your ability to relax*' and your ability to relax is governed by how effective your trusted system is at capturing and containing everything. He gives the analogy of having a 'mind like water'. When a pebble is thrown into the water, the water ripples, absorbing the force of the pebble, and then returns to a position of calm. This is how we need to endeavour to be at work. The trusted system is this starting point. If everything is in your system you have a clear view of what there is to do. In my example above the student asking to see me at the end of lecture is such a 'pebble'. By having a trusted system, I know what there is to do next and later and can decide what options I can offer the student based on that system. The same applies when your manager drops a task on you. You can use your trusted system to show you have the time, or not, or move things around quickly and safely, knowing you won't forget anything. This will accommodate the new challenge, and then return you to a state of calm.

Once you have a trusted system, you're ready to go!

Keeping your trusted system up to date

Remember the trusted system is an all or nothing system so everything needs to go in there. It's maybe not physically possible or appropriate to update the trusted system as you are going through the day so we need some method of collecting things that we can then transfer into our trusted system frequently. You need to use something, or some things, that you have easy access to. It doesn't really matter how many methods you use to catch your tasks but the less you have the better. You just need to have enough methods to cover the scenarios you work in. The secret is to empty the places you have caught things in regularly. I use the 'notes' feature on my smartphone and a notebook that lives on my desk or in my bag. Other things are also catching tasks for you. No doubt you will have voicemail on your phone, you may well receive written correspondence, and you will certainly receive emails. We will look at emails specifically later in the chapter as they are both an asset and a curse. Wherever you catch tasks you need to 'empty' these into your trusted system regularly. I do this at the end of every day, or if I'm away from my desk at the end of the day, I do it first thing the following morning.

Single tasking

Once we know what there is to do how do we set about doing it? As we have seen above multitasking has its problems. Single tasking is a much more effective approach. Single tasking relies on having planned your day. You cannot effectively plan and do at the same time so by planning in one phase of your day and doing in another you improve your productivity. Wilson explored the impact of knowing you had an unopened email on productivity and showed that simply thinking about multitasking by reading the email reduced IQ by ten points (Levitin, 2015). Single tasking requires you to engage in one task to the exclusion of all other tasks. For example, I now deal with my emails at strategic points during the day and when I'm not working on emails, I close down my email client so that I get no 'pop up' message when I get an email. Just knowing the email is there even if I don't go to read it draws on my psychological capacity to stay on task. In order to single task we need a clear view of what there is to do, we need to plan how to do it and then engage in the doing, one task at a time. Engaging our deliberate system so we can plan and organise means we handle the day, rather than the day handling us. If we only work with our automatic system, tacking tasks in a haphazard way, we will make poor decisions based on gut reactions. Our deliberate system is where our reasoning and analysis and forward thinking take place. There's more about our automatic and deliberate brain on page 128.

When we engage this system with the non-routine we start to clarify what we are presented with and what we need to do with it (Kahneman, 2011; Webb, 2017). Webb (2017) says that with our deliberate system engaged we will:

* review information;
* connect it to past experience;
* make sense of it;
* generate options;
* evaluate options.

In doing this you will think about your future work (later today, next week and even next year) and consider how to get there by thinking about the benefits of certain courses of action. Planning like this is bringing the future into the present so you can have a good long look it (Lakein, 1974).

Chunking

Once we have planned, we can start 'chunking' tasks together. By batching or chunking similar tasks together you are engaging your brain in a particular way of thinking rather than switching between different modes of operation. This way you can apply yourself fully to particular types of task by utilising a single attentional set. As Levitin (2015, p 175) puts it, *'if you have chores to do, put similar chores together'*. If you are like me, you will have experienced this while reading. I find it difficult to read while the TV is on in the background, but equally on an evening I like to sit with my wife. She isn't a reader. When I start to read under these circumstances, I find my reading slow and laborious, and I keep being distracted by the TV. But then something magical happens. Unconsciously the TV fades into the background and I start to focus on what I'm reading, and my reading speed quickens. If I switch and go into the kitchen to prepare the evening meal, when I come back to reading I will have to start again to set my attention. Task switching has an attentional cost to it.

It's useful to start thinking about how you will 'chunk' tasks by considering the general aspects of your job role and identifying broad categories of things you are asked to do or skills you are asked to utilise. I tried this for my job and came up with the following:

- emails (I really feel you need to keep this as a task all on its own);
- having conversations (meetings, telephone calls, lectures);
- reading and researching;
- writing;
- planning (which also needs to be an element on its own).

Once you have this list you need to think about periods of time when you can batch all of the tasks that fit into these categories together as far as is practicable. I appreciate that some things you do simply have to happen at certain times of day, so that may be unavoidable. For me, lectures are scheduled so I can't move those. But what I can do is schedule similar tasks around those fixed tasks. Once you have your list of task types and a list of tasks group them together into allocated times avoiding switching between the task groups (Webb, 2017).

So, a typical lecturing day for me would look like this:

8.00 to 8.30	planning
8.30 to 9.00	emails
9.00 to 10.00	having conversations (tutorials, meetings, discussions with colleagues)
10.00 to 12.00	having conversations (lecturing)
12.00 to 12.30	lunch
12.30 to 13.00	emails
13.00 to 15.00	having conversations (lecturing)
15.00 to 16.00	reading and researching (documents that have been emailed to me, lecture preparation)
16.00 to 16.30	emails
16.30 to 17.00	planning.

On a day when I'm not lecturing I can 'chunk' even more effectively. The larger the 'chunks' the better:

8.00 to 8.30	planning
8.30 to 9.00	emails
9.00 to 12.00	reading and researching (documents that have been emailed to me, lecture preparation, study)
12.00 to 12.30	lunch
12.30 to 13.00	emails
13.00 to 15.00	writing (writing lectures, reports, long-form responses)
15.00 to 16.00	having conversations (tutorials, meetings, discussions with colleagues)
16.00 to 16.30	emails
16.30 to 17.00	planning.

Obviously, depending on the tasks you need to do, these times move around, but you can get a sense of the idea.

Timing is everything

When thinking about where to chunk specific work tasks you may want to consider your chronotype. While we all follow a broadly 24-hour pattern of waking and sleeping we all have peaks and troughs that are unique to ourselves. We need to understand our chronotype to know when we are at our best for various tasks. If, like me, you are a morning type then you should schedule your complex thinking tasks early in the day. I have a slump around 11am and then a further peak from about 1.30pm to 3pm. After 3pm I'm no good for anything! I can't just stop work at 3pm so what I do is schedule routine administrative tasks that take little thinking about. You will need to think about whether you are like me, a lark, or whether you are more of a night owl who takes time to get going on a morning but is completely fired up in the afternoon. By scheduling tasks that complement your chronotype you will be more productive (Walker, 2018).

Think about your chronotype. When are you at your most alert? When are you most focused? When do you have a productivity 'dip'?

Write a list of all of your tasks at work.

Group these tasks together into tasks that require a similar way of using your brain.

Think about what time of day would be best for you to complete these 'chunks' of tasks based on your chronotype.

Emails: an asset and a curse

How many of you have inboxes with hundreds if not thousands of emails in them? I suspect most of you. What happens to the emails that have disappeared off the bottom of the screen? The answer is they seldom get looked at until someone asks for something and says they emailed you about it. Then you might have a look and there it is! This type of incident erodes your professional status among your peers.

Your email inbox is for collecting things that you need to do something with and is not a long-term storage solution. Your inbox should be emptied daily. You should empty it first when you are creating your trusted system and then it should be emptied by the end of every day after that. Allen (2015) gives us an easy to remember process telling us you should look at each email and either:

do it,

delegate it,

defer it, or

delete it.

Use these four steps to empty your inbox. Let's look at these each in turn.

Do it! That's it – just do it. Read the email, figure out what's in it to do and just do it. Here we apply the two-minute rule (Allen, 2015). The two-minute rule is an excellent way to get things done. Earlier we noted that the planning fallacy leads us to think that small tasks take longer than they do. The rule here is if it going to take less than two minutes to do then you just do it. Don't put it off, don't put it into your trusted system, just do it. You'll work through many emails using this two-minute rule method, I'm sure. You'll quickly get a feel for what can be achieved in two minutes, and it's probably more than you think. Note, though, this rule doesn't just apply to emails but can be applied to everything in your life. You will be amazed at how much just gets done.

While you are going through your emails and identifying your 'do it' tasks, employ the 'delete it' process. Think, '*Is this anything to do with me? Do I need to do anything with it? Has someone copied me into something that I don't need to know about or keep?*' Or, '*I've read it using the two-minute rule and now I'm done with it.*' If you think you might need it later, set yourself up a reference folder and move it there. Remember we're trying to get our inbox empty.

While you are going through your emails doing or deleting you can also be delegating. Delegating is not a top down idea. Yes, managers delegate to their team but delegation is also about you identifying that you need a decision or advice from your manager – upward delegation – or you need to consult with a colleague – sideways delegation. Either way the point is that you can't respond until you have something from someone else. Once you've asked that someone else for what you want you are done with this email. You might be brave enough to delete it – for example if a student asks me for availability to meet, I'll email some dates back and delete the email because the ball is back in their court. If I think I might need to refer to the email later, I file it in a folder. I periodically empty my deleted items folder once they are two weeks old as by that point someone should have been back to me if it was that important.

Finally, once we've done all of that, we get to the emails that are going to need more of our attention. These are the ones that need us to undertake a task ourselves. Remembering that we are endeavouring to empty our inbox, we need to use our trusted system and put all of our tasks into it. So, things like *'Meet Jane on 17th Feb at 2 in Room 321 for appraisal'* go into a timeslot. I use the 'all day' event section for items that I want to get done but aren't specific to a time and date at the moment. So, for now, I'll put *'Draft report for meeting on the 12th June'* as an all-day event. I'll put *'Complete report for meeting on 12th June'* in as an event the week before the 12th of June to remind me to finish the report. This will eventually become time specific as I'll have to set time aside to do it but, as long as it's still a while off, it can sit in a day where I think I might get it done and if I don't I can move it into another day until it becomes critical to do it. This way you don't lose anything. If there's no time frame – for example, *'Jane has asked me think about conferences I might want to attend next year'* – then that goes in the spreadsheet for later consideration.

SO, LET'S GET STARTED: IT'S MONDAY MORNING

No, no, stop. Rewind. Go back.

Having a good Monday at work (or whatever day your first day back is) starts with what you did at the end of the last day you were at work. So, for the majority of us, what you did at the end of Friday will have more impact on your Monday than what you do at the start of Monday. *'Planning and doing require separate parts of the brain'*, so we need to do them at different times (Levitin, 2015, p 174). The risk of leaving all of your planning for the week ahead until Monday morning is that if something urgent is required when you arrive at work, you will fall into planning and doing at the same time because you will deprioritise the planning.

My week starts with 30 to 45 minutes on a Friday afternoon when I plan the following week and look ahead, sometimes up to three weeks to a month ahead. Knowing what's coming helps you set up the environment to support productivity. Remember, planning brings the future into the present so that you can explore it and think about it (Lakein, 1974).

This Friday afternoon ritual happens because it is in my diary as a recurring event. Along with 30 minutes on a morning every day and 30 minutes on an afternoon every day. Sometimes I use all of this time, sometimes only a little of it, but by putting it in my diary it remains protected and is only moved or deleted if absolutely necessary. When I do decide to delete it and not do it, I can do this, safe in the knowledge that because I get my inbox to empty every day, there can be nothing lurking in there that's more than a few hours old. This helps me leave that behind and focus on the pressing task that was so important I was happy to give up my planning time. Note, though, tomorrow morning's planning time has now become doubly important.

I look ahead to next week and work through each day. I have a folder marked up with each of the days of the week and if I need to print anything I print it on a Friday afternoon and put it into the day in the folder. My folder works two weeks ahead, so I do the same for the following week as well. I go through the tasks in my calendar one at a time and do a number of things as well as the printing. I ask myself *'Have I got all of the information available that I need for that calendar event?'* Sometimes that's room numbers for teaching, addresses for visits I need to do, names of people I'm visiting, phone numbers for people I need to call. If these aren't already there in my calendar, I find them and put them there so when I get to that task next week what I need is already available to me.

While I'm doing this, I'm looking at time and date specific events and the 'all day' events in my calendar that may be becoming time and date specific. If they are then I move them into a slot in my calendar, remembering to 'chunk' similar tasks together and give myself enough time for each task. Remember, overestimating is better than underestimating when it comes to setting time aside.

As I work through my calendar and I find an end date for a bigger task, then I explore breaking this task down into smaller steps. This is why it is crucial to work several weeks ahead during your Friday planning session, as if you only work a week ahead you will probably find only limited amounts of time in your schedule to do this. The further you work ahead the less chance there is of something creeping up on you.

DEALING WITH BIG TASKS, OR, HOW DO YOU EAT AN ELEPHANT?

How do you eat an elephant? One bite at a time… so the joke goes. Elephants are simply too big to eat all in one sitting! If you were going to run a marathon you wouldn't get up one day and give it a go. You'd break the big task down into manageable smaller tasks in order to get to the end result. If you were going to build a house, you'd start with the idea of what the finished house would look like and then break it down into tasks that you need to achieve to move towards building the house. If you had to find the time to build a house, you'd be hard pushed to fit it into your diary in one chunk but if you were to break it down into tasks that fit into a weekend and then work on those tasks each weekend you'd eventually build a house. This relies on an idea called the power of small wins. The brain's reward system gives you a neurochemical hit every time you complete a task (Levitin, 2015; Webb, 2017). If your task is to write a chapter of a book, you will only get that positive, feel-good spike when you write the chapter of the book. But, if you break that down into research books to read, read relevant chapters, make notes from books, write a plan for the chapter, write the first section, write the second section, proofread the chapter, send the chapter to the publisher, then you will get a 'feel-good' rush when you achieve each step and 'tick it off' your calendar. This helps maintain your motivation towards completion of the task and makes each element feel doable and much easier to fit into the gaps in your calendar.

You need to define the starting point, the initiating task, because making a start is the hardest part, so planning how to start is crucial. You also need to define what the end product looks like and when it needs to done by. Then in between you diary the steps that are required to get you from A to B. Sometimes I find that, as I'm planning, some of the smaller tasks in themselves feel quite onerous, so I break those down into smaller tasks. You can then diary these separately or sometimes I'll break them down in the notes section of the calendar event. As Allen (2015) says, you can't plan and do. So do the planning first, then when you hit the task in your calendar you can just get on with the doing, step by step.

SO, IS IT MONDAY MORNING YET?

It is indeed! If you got your planning right on Friday, hopefully that gave you a sense of what there was to do this week, you got all your plans in place, and went home satisfied that you could leave work at work, safe in the knowledge it would be all there waiting for you, neat and tidy and sorted ready for you to start. Leaving the job behind on a Friday is difficult but being methodical about your planning and organisation does help to relieve stress (Allen, 2015). The purpose of being organised is to give psychological capacity and the ability to 'leave behind'.

Here's what my Monday looks like (in fact here's what every morning looks like!).

- Make coffee!
- Open up computer.
- Open up diary and read through 'today', having a quick glance at the rest of the week. It should all look familiar as you only looked at it on Friday (or the previous working day).
- Open up spreadsheet and have a quick glance through it. Again, there should be no surprises in there as you only looked at it the previous working day but doing this reacquaints you with your trusted system.
- Check I have everything available to me for the events in my calendar for today. You should have as you dealt with this the previous working day but checking helps you confirm all is well and switch off from it to concentrate on other things. You are reassured.
- Open up emails.
- Get inbox to empty (do it, defer it, delegate it, delete it). Starting your day by reacquainting yourself with your trusted system should make it easier to 'defer' things into it as you will know where the gaps, or non-essential tasks, are that can be moved.
- Close down email client. (Personally I check my emails again in the middle and at the end of the day and generally not in between. Remember switching between tasks is distracting and impacts negatively on our productivity.)

Start on tasks for the day – always eating any frogs first.

EAT THAT FROG

What's the worst thing you can think of to do? Well, it might be to eat a live frog. As this old adage attributed to Mark Twain goes – if the worst thing you had to do at the start of the day was eat a live frog, once you'd done it, there'd not be much else in your day that would be worse. So, eat that frog! Do the worst thing first. What things in your email, or in your diary, are going to diminish your psychological capital all day if they remain undone? I've spent many a day getting nothing done because that difficult phone call still needs making, or that problematic email needs a response, or that information I need that will be really difficult to get hold of hasn't been dealt with. Such things keep popping into your head while you are trying to do other things. Tracy (2017, p 2) offers us this advice for 'eating frogs': '*If you have to eat a live frog at all, it doesn't pay to sit and look at it for very long*', and, '*If you have to eat two frogs eat the ugliest one first.*' Get on with it and do the worst thing first. Once you've dealt with these difficult tasks you will be psychologically free of them to get on with your day.

THE END OF THE DAY: PRIORITISING FOR TOMORROW AND BEYOND

So, you planned your week on Friday, you checked and planned your day in the morning, and you've spent all day working on your tasks. You will now have emails in your inbox, notes you've made during the day and voicemails. It's time to get 'in' to 'empty' again. It doesn't matter what order you do things in but while working through the things that have been captured in various places employ this 'now, next, noted and never' method.

- **Now**: You will come across things that you can simply do by utilising the two-minute rule and you will come across things that are urgent. You may have capacity or may need to do these things now. It pays not to leave your end of day planning until the absolute end of the day as you may come across something that simply needs to be dealt with. If you need to get away from the office by a particular time, do your planning a little earlier. Other 'now' things might be ok to be left until the morning. Put them in your calendar for the next day in a time slot.
- **Next**: Your next things will be less urgent. They will need to be done soon but they don't need to be done as soon as possible. They need to be done 'next' once your 'now' things are done. Figure out a time scale, diary the end goal, break it down into steps, identify a start point and diary those. You need to know what you're aiming for and what the steps are to get there before you can set when you will start.
- **Noted**: There will be things you've identified that are simply interesting things to note. Maybe something you want to read, or a website to look at when you have time, or an idea that needs developing. Most of these go into my spreadsheet but sometimes I'll put them in my calendar as an all-day event in a day that looks fairly free. If by the time I get to that day the day isn't fairly free anymore I can just move whatever it is to the next week and have another go at trying to look at it then.

- **Never:** Finally, you will have been sent emails that contain things that you've looked at and dismissed, so delete them. You may have written something down and on reflection you don't want to go any further with it so cross it out. You may need to use the two-minute rule to say no to something. If it's 'never', it's 'never', so get rid of it.

Then, look at the next day and make sure you have everything you need to hand to make it a productive day. Eventually you are back to Friday (or your last working day of the week) and you are planning next week and next month. This perpetual cycle keeps you focused on your tasks and reassures you regularly that all is in order. It gives you frequent opportunities to reconsider priorities and opportunities to ensure that you are making the best use of the time you have available to you. Making the best use of your time leads to being more productive. We've looked at applying these strategies to work here but they work equally as well in planning your personal life. Don't tell my friends but they are all on my spreadsheet with when I plan to see them next!

REMEMBER THESE KEY THINGS

- Knowing what to do is about knowing what you can safely not do.
- Optimise your day by chunking similar tasks together.
- Today starts the day before.
- Eat your frogs as soon as you can... and don't look at them for too long.
- Break big tasks into smaller tasks to get a motivation buzz from small wins.
- Everything we've talked about is habit forming but it is likely to feel like hard work for the first few months till it becomes part of how you work.
- Plan effectively – never 'touch' things twice – and do something while it's on your mind.
- Don't get distracted. Only check emails at designated times and go 'off the grid' in between checking.
- Get the technology to work for you. Need to focus on a report and you have two hours before a meeting? Set a reminder on your phone 15 minutes before the meeting to stop you checking the time and interrupting your flow ... and to make sure you don't miss the meeting.

REFERENCES

Allen, D (2015) *Getting Things Done: The Art of Stress-free Productivity*. London: Piatkus.

Dux, P E, Ivanoff, J, Asplund, C L and Marois, R (2006) Isolation of a Central Bottleneck of Information Processing with Time Resolved fMRI. *Neuron*, 52(6): 1109–20.

Heylighen, F and Vidal, C (2007) Getting Things Done: The Science behind Stress-free Productivity. Brussels: Evolution, Complexity and Cognition Research Group (Free University of Brussels).

Iqbal, S T and Horvitz, E (2007) Disruption and Recovery of Computing Tasks: Field Study, Analysis, and Directions. Paper presented at CHI 2007, 28 April–3 May 2007, San Jose, CA.

Kahneman, D (2011) *Thinking, Fast and Slow*. London: Penguin.

Keller, G and Papasan, J (2014) *The One Thing*. London: John Murray.

Lakein, A (1974) *How to Get Control of Your Time and Your Life*. London: Signet.

Levitin, D (2015) *The Organized Mind: Thinking Straight in the Age of Information Overload*. London: Penguin.

Tracy, B (2017) *Eat That Frog*. London: Hodder and Stoughton.

Walker, M (2018) *Why We Sleep*. London: Penguin Random House.

Webb, C (2017) *How to Have a Good Day: The Essential Toolkit for a Productive Day at Work and Beyond*. London: Palgrave Macmillan.

Wray, S and Rymell, S (2014) Personal Organization and Time Management. In Grant, L and Kinman, G (eds) *Developing Resilience for Social Work Practice* (pp 73–92). London: Palgrave.

8 Finding your motivation mojo: making a start's the hardest part

Stephen

HOW TO START AND HOW TO KEEP GOING

You know how this goes. You know you need to get on with the task, yet you find yourself rearranging the paperwork on your desk or tidying your stationery drawer. You know the deadline is looming, but you find yourself distracted, checking your emails or your Twitter feed. You find yourself making coffee, sometimes for the whole office. You find yourself chatting to a colleague. Yet you know there is something pressing that needs to be done. So why do you not get on and do it?! I'm confident to say this is a problem for us all. Motivating yourself to get started – or 'making a start is the hardest part', as I'm fond of saying to my wife, which doesn't annoy her at all – can be difficult. Then, keeping going once you've started, with all the distractions that modern life and the modern workplace have to throw at us, can be just as difficult. Finally, tidying up all the loose ends and getting the job finished, my own nemesis, can get lost in the distraction of starting other things.

ARE WE READY FOR THIS 'FUTURE'?

Written in 1970, Alvin Toffler's *Futureshock* uncannily predicted the world we now live in. This world that underpins some of the problems we face. He observed this:

> *In the three short decades between now* [1970] *and the twenty-first century, millions of ordinary, psychologically normal* [sic] *people will face an abrupt collision with the future. Citizens of the world's richest and most technologically advanced nations, many of them will find it increasingly painful to keep up with the incessant demand for change that characterizes our time. For them, the future will have arrived too soon.*
>
> (Toffler, 1970, p 9)

He goes on to talk about the death of permanence and an ever-changing world that we are simply not, from an evolutionary perspective, ready for. We have developed a world that is always connected, featuring a constant stream of distractions that can divert our attention to the trivial and away from the important. This has the impact of sapping our desire and motivation to get on with the essential and then creates stress when we have wasted time but still have important things to do and not enough time to do them. I'm sure many of us have disappeared down a Facebook 'rabbit hole', emerging half an hour or more later wondering what just happened.

In terms of technological development, those born in the early part of the twentieth century were born at the median point of human progress. The world now, in the twenty-first century, compared to the early part of the twentieth century, is as far removed from that time as that time was from the period of Julius Caesar's reign (Toffler, 1970). We can't keep up. How do we remain focused and motivated on the task in hand when we are on shifting sands, constantly distracted and often overwhelmed by information onslaught?

THE MODERN WORKPLACE

These social and technological changes permeate the workplace, which is often now a place of constant transformation. What 'was' last month often 'isn't' this month. Cannon (2018) points out the significance of work in an adult's life. The significance that binds us to this ever changing environment. She identifies not only that it gives us socio-economic status (and helps us pay the bills!) but also that it gives us a sense of achievement, success and pride. It can fuel our self-esteem or has the potential to degrade it. We spend a lot of time at work so the working environment we find ourselves in has the capacity to have a huge impact on us. For social workers, and indeed other professionals who are person facing, our careers are often more than just a job. There is a motivating energy in what could be considered a 'calling'. This 'calling energy' can lead to enthusiasm, self-starting and motivation. This internal energy drives us when we are happy, enthusiastic and loving what we do (Jaeger, 2004). Yet still we are prone to procrastination.

Work has become very different for many. It has moved from being about trading time for money in order to survive into a vocation that generates a better life outside of work. It encourages career growth through enjoyable developmental activities during work time (Pradhan et al, 2017). The working environment can keep us engaged, and therefore motivated, by creating alignment between meaning derived from work and a person's interests. The culture of the organisation and the organisation's priorities need to be 'in tune' with people's personal interests. When they are, '*employees want to come to work*', and when they aren't, '*problems rise to the surface*' (Taylor, 2015, p 28). When there is this link, a person's professional identity is formed (Pradhan et al, 2017). In a profession like social work this professional identity influences and correlates with personal identity. These connections fuel passion for the job and therefore fuel motivation.

As a lecturer in a university I get the pleasure of talking to students about their motivation to be social workers. I also come into contact with many practitioners and can talk to them about the same. One of the things we often talk about at interview for places on the course is what has motivated the applicant to apply to undertake the qualification to become a social worker. They gush with enthusiasm and talk about making a difference in people's lives, supporting people through crises, being a good listener and promoting social justice. They also talk about what they will get from it: a sense of pride in a job well done, a sense of pleasure for themselves in seeing people develop and emerge from difficulties, and the sense of achievement of professional status born out of studying.

While I don't think these motivators leave qualified practitioners, they seem, after a time, to lurk only in the background. I observe a shift from being motivated by internal drivers, things they want for themselves, to being externally motivated by court dates, end dates on reports, making sure the right numbers of visits are made, and making sure the boxes are ticked and the process completed. These are all necessary and fundamental things to doing the job but they are not why people entered the profession and not what will ultimately motivate them effectively.

INTRINSIC AND EXTRINSIC MOTIVATION

From the dawning of the industrial revolution, how to motivate people at work has been given serious consideration. Thinking quickly moved beyond salary as a motivator to broader considerations. Elton Musk (1880–1949) identified that attention needed to be given to emotional responses and the social climate in workplaces (Coulshed and Mullender, 2006). Chris Argyris (1923–2013) noted that where people had little control over their work initiative was lacking and resistance to change was evident (Argyris, 1957). Douglas McGregor (1906–64) felt that people naturally strive, want to take pride in their work and seek new experiences (McGregor, 1960). He noted that people thrive best in organisations where they are delegated control and responsibility.

DOUGLAS MCGREGOR AND MOTIVATION

In the 1960s, social psychologist Douglas McGregor developed two ideas that he called 'Theory X' and 'Theory Y' to explain how the view of managers regarding what motivated staff affected their management style.

Theory X

Theory X suggests that people need a 'carrot and stick' approach to motivate them. External rewards (the carrot) or direct motivation through the threat of punishment (the stick) are what motivates. This idea suggests that people generally dislike work and need constant direction as they will not take responsibility for themselves. They need to be micromanaged every step of the way. Workers are generally not ambitious, and their general position is one of a lack of motivation.

Managers who view workers like this feel the need to set targets, often based around numbers of things done or outputs achieved, much like performance indicators. Organisations that view workers like this tend to have a hierarchical structure of tiers of managers. Authority and control reside in the managers and such structures and attitudes tend to dominate in environments that employ large numbers of people where working to tight deadlines is required.

Theory Y

Theory Y suggests that people like to work on their own initiative and be self-motivated towards completing tasks. People view work positively as a fulfilling activity and want to take ownership of their work. Workers want to be involved in decision making. This reflects a desire in workers to have a meaningful career and not simply be 'a cog in the machine'.

Managers who view workers in this way have a more participative management style more akin to leadership. They collaborate and trust the views of their team more. They pass on some control and responsibility to their team and encourage open communication.

Are you more like a Theory X or Theory Y worker?

Does your organisation view you like a Theory X or Theory Y worker?

Are workers more like Theory Y workers while organisations use methods more in line with Theory X to motivate?

When someone sets their goals from their personal value perspective and considers what they want to achieve for themselves from an internal viewpoint they are being internally or intrinsically motivated. For social workers it might be '*I want to support people to exercise their rights as rights are important to me*', or, '*I want to do a good job and utilise my skills and knowledge*'. Intrinsic motivators fuel behaviour that is enjoyable and purposeful and provides sufficient motivation that people persist in undertaking the task (Cerasoli et al, 2014). Intrinsic motivation is born out of engaging in something personally rewarding.

Extrinsic motivation relies on rewards or the desire to avoid punishment. We are rewarded for doing our job with a salary or we avoid the 'punishment' of a reprimand by our manager by getting that report done on time. There is not a simple straightforward binary here that defines intrinsic as good and extrinsic as bad, although, as we shall see, intrinsic motivators in the social work job role are more likely to promote motivation and job satisfaction while mitigating stress. Extrinsic rewards do have their place. Incentives (things like bonuses for example) were shown to produce a 22 per cent increase in performance but largely in manual work rather than cognitive work (Taylor, 2015). Pink (2018) suggests that extrinsic motivators like salary have their limits and explains that once someone has enough money to achieve a good standard of living paying them more doesn't necessarily result in enhanced motivation. In fact, he notes that further extrinsic rewards can actually demotivate. With simple, measurable tasks a direct incentive can motivate, whereas where teamwork and creativity is required incentives can undermine intrinsic motivation and have been shown to encourage counterproductive behaviours (Pink, 2018; Taylor, 2015).

> *Work consists of whatever a body is obliged to do. Play consists of whatever a body is not obliged to do.*
>
> Mark Twain (2011 [1876])

In *The Adventures of Tom Sawyer*, originally published in 1876, Twain creates a scene in which Tom is painting Aunt Polly's fence. Obviously, Tom wishes he could play instead of having to do this chore, which is punishment for his misbehaviour. One of his friends, Ben, sees him doing this 'work' and pokes fun at him for having to do it. In response Tom says, *'This ain't work?'* He proceeds to carefully and precisely paint the fence. *'You don't get to do this every day'*, he says to Ben. *'Let me paint a little'*, Ben says to Tom. *'Aunt Polly says this is so important only Tom Sawyer can do it'*, says Tom. Ben can't resist such an important thing and even offers Tom his apple in exchange for a chance to paint. Other boys come along as Ben paints the fence and offer Tom various things for the thrill of getting involved.

Motivation is everything. How you approach a task impacts on how you view the task.

The Sawyer effect

Pink (2018) recounts an experiment in which children were asked to draw. They were divided into three groups. The first group were shown a certificate they would be given after they had drawn and were asked if they wanted to draw in order to receive it. The second group were asked if they wanted to draw and were not offered anything for doing so. They were then given a certificate after they had drawn. The final group were asked if they wanted to draw and after doing so were given nothing.

Two weeks later the same groups were asked if they wanted to draw again. The second and third groups engaged just as much as they had the first time while the group who had expected and received an award showed much less interest.

Pink refers to this as the 'Sawyer effect'. Play has been turned into work for the first group. This he suggests is the impact if the *'if you do this then you get this'* phenomenon which generates an extrinsic motivation rather than the intrinsic, *'I want to draw because I enjoy drawing'* of the other two groups.

SELF-DETERMINATION THEORY

To consider how intrinsic motivation works we should explore the dominant theory in this area, which is self-determination theory. Developed by Deci and Ryan, it explains how *'intrinsic motivation fuels the direction, intensity, and persistence of motivated behaviour'* (Cerasoli et al, 2014, p 982). The theory suggests that we have three innate psychological needs, autonomy, competence (or mastery) and interconnectedness (Pink, 2018).

The suggestion is that when we cannot satisfy these needs our productivity, motivation, and therefore our happiness, reduce. Pink (2018) comments that we enter this world as children wired to be active and engaged, ready to explore and develop, but somehow later on we can become passive. He argues that in the workplace it can be how we are managed that switches us to this state because of how we are asked to work. It is being motivated extrinsically rather than intrinsically that is causing the problem.

The first element, autonomy, can be difficult to achieve in some settings. Some things simply have to be done when they have to be done, there is no choice. This is not the case in social work. While 'end dates' and 'court dates' are still persistent motivators, how you get to those dates is largely in your hands. As a practitioner you have control over the order in which you approach tasks, how you approach them and sometimes which tasks to undertake. Research has shown that giving people a sense of autonomy leads to '*higher productivity, less burnout, and greater levels of psychological well-being*' (Pink, 2018, p 91). When social workers are motivated by extrinsic motivators they are less likely to be happy workers. But, Pink (2018) observes, when workers are given autonomy to control their work we see the improvements. Managers, take note.

The second element that fuels motivation is that of mastery. Mastering something takes time and requires direct attention to the task. This requires the right sort of working environment where people have the time to reflect. Reflection forms a crucial part of the process of learning and mastering. Mastering also requires good quality feedback and the place for this is in supervision. Supervision for qualified practitioners should be the same as supervision for students. It should not simply be about cases but should be about development, not to mention emotions. Mastery also relies on the individual creating the right working environment for themselves and on the internal order that self-care and being organised seek to create. Trying to work amidst chaos does not promote motivation. The 'being organised' chapter (Chapter 7) will assist with ideas for this to help you stay on task without being distracted, to single task not multitask, and to have a system to control the things external to you. The application of these ideas and tools can create calm in the moment so that you can dedicate yourself to mastering what is at hand. Mastery enhances concentration, which enhances 'flow', which enhances productivity. And, as a wonderful bonus, it makes people happy (Newport, 2016).

For the final element, that of interconnectedness, Pink (2018) translates this into purpose. Non-monetary motivators, as we have seen, are becoming increasingly important to people. Purpose comes from this mindset, from internal values. Social work is all about purpose and about interconnectedness. Working alongside colleagues, other professionals, families, service users and carers connects us to real-world, real-life concerns. This purpose, both sited outside and beyond yourself and constructed internally, is a powerful force to motivate. We are left with the position that intrinsic motivation, in the person-focused work we do, is more important than extrinsic motivation. Being motivated by and for the people we work with is more important, in terms of motivation and mitigation of stress, than the date the report is due. It is important to reflect regularly on this to connect yourself to this motivating force.

WHAT IS GETTING IN THE WAY?

Procrastination

Getting going can be difficult at times. Using some of the ideas in the chapter on being organised (Chapter 7) will help. Things like the 'two-minute rule' and 'how to eat an elephant' are useful. Chipping away at tasks by deconstructing them into smaller tasks helps to get going. But no matter how hard we try, we sometimes find ourselves stuck, shuffling papers, not knowing where to start and reaching for the kettle instead of the next essential task. Motivating ourselves to get going can be problematic. Sometimes we simply avoid the task altogether. Avoidance is the successful removal of the thing we don't want to do from the here and now. The problem with this is the task still remains there to be done. Our desire to avoid or tackle a task is often rooted in how motivated we are to achieve the task and, as we have seen, how motivated we are is rooted in whether the motivation is extrinsic – a motivational factor external to us – or intrinsic – a motivational factor generated internally.

Steel (in Levitin, 2015) says we procrastinate because, in the moment, we have a low tolerance for frustration – so if something appears difficult, we will tend to put it off. When we do initiate a task, we tend to choose the easiest tasks rather than the ones that will give us the greatest reward in the long term. He suggests that there are two problems with the human mind. First, we think life should be easy, so we have a tendency to put off difficult things and, second, our self-worth is bound up in our success. If something looks like it is going to be difficult and there's a risk we might not do it well then we put off doing it. There's an obvious link here to Deci and Ryan's idea of mastery that we've just considered. My nemesis was always difficult conversations with family members of service users I worked with. I don't like conflict and my preference is for people to like me, so I would put off conversations where I had a difficult message to relay that might result in me not being liked and somehow feeling that I had failed. I have spent all day at times getting nothing done, worrying about conversations, concentrating my efforts on low value tasks, only to find when I had the conversation it went well. What a waste! I should have eaten that frog!

Levitin (2015) recounts Steel's equation for procrastination. If we are confident with the task and the value of the task is high, we are less likely to procrastinate. Working against these factors are two others: how long it will take to complete the task and how easily we are distracted. If it's a short task and we are not easily distracted, then we won't procrastinate (this is where the two-minute rule is effective). But, when things are the other way around and it is a long task, and there are things available to us to distract us, then we may find ourselves putting off getting started (this is why you should shut your email down when trying to work on tasks). The reality is, when confronted with a list of tasks, we are more likely to get on with the trivial than launch ourselves into a high value but more complex task (Tracy, 2017). In a sense, our psychological make up conspires against us, as we get a psychological buzz whenever we complete a task. Completing low value, short tasks creates the illusion of getting on with things, and sometimes there's no harm in getting some of those small tasks done – but you need to be aware that you are potentially storing up a problem for later by not making a start on more complex tasks.

The secret is to block out some time to do all of the small tasks, so they are done before embarking on a long task. This effectively turns lots of small tasks into one big task of *'getting my small tasks done'*.

This is why Allen (2015) says that traditional 'to do' lists made once we hit a crisis point don't work. Firstly, you are never sure you have captured everything on your 'to do' list, which is why he prefers the concept of a 'trusted system', and secondly you will pick easy tasks not difficult ones. How many of us find old 'to do' lists only to discover things still not done? This problem of not starting complex tasks, even when we know we really should, is why the suggestion to break large tasks down into small ones works well. When the task looks achievable, we are more likely to feel we have the time and skill, the mastery, to achieve it (this is where using the 'how to eat an elephant' trick works). The longer you put off that difficult, time consuming task, the less time you will have to complete it. As Benjamin Franklin reputedly said, *'You may delay, but time will not'*.

Our lazy brain

One of the other problems here is we have what is referred to as 'present bias'. This is the tendency to want something that makes us feel good now rather than delay gratification and have something that makes us feel good later. We prefer to turn to things that are readily available rather than put the effort in to engage our brains and do something difficult. This is a hangover from our evolutionary history; dealing with things quickly, in the moment, for our primitive ancestors – running away from a dangerous wild animal, for example – was far more important than thinking about later benefits (Webb, 2017). To understand this, we need to look at how the brain works.

Kahneman (2011) proposes that we have two systems at work in our brain: the fast system and the slow system. Webb (2017) calls these the automatic system and the deliberate system. The fast, or automatic, system works like this. Whenever we need to respond to something, we are inclined towards an automatic pre-programmed response. These responses are usually based on our instincts – the fight, flight, or freeze response, for example. We are confronted with hostility and, without thinking, we move away, or we retaliate. These responses are not thought through. They exist in our subconscious and it's a good thing they are there. They help us get on with driving our car, while thinking about the day ahead or chatting to our passenger. Much of what we need to do to drive safely is automated once we become experienced. It is so ingrained in us that we are unaware that our subconscious is taking care of things. If someone steps out in front of you, you will react but until that point of reaction you will not have been consciously aware of all the things going on with your driving. The problem is that our automatic system is not very clever. It tends to filter and sift without looking at the detail. In order to start thinking deeply we need to engage our slow or deliberate system, and this is hard work. So, we opt for the easy task or procrastinate delaying the start of the difficult task. Generally, putting off something that is in some way difficult will leave you worse off when you come to need to do it (Ainslie, 2010).

Levitin (2015, p 196) makes it clear that procrastination is *'a failure of self-regulation, planning, impulse control, or a combination of all three. By definition, it involves us delaying an activity, task, or decision that would help us reach our goals.*' Without conscious planning we leave our daily responses open to automatic thinking rather than deliberate thinking, and we end up doing the task that 'shouts the loudest' rather than the one that clear planning would have led us to conclude really was our priority.

> *If you fail to plan, you are planning to fail.*
> Benjamin Franklin

Motivation is finite

Motivation relies on us being disciplined and exploring tasks in a structured way. Anyone who has ever been on a diet knows that the resilience of our being motivated towards a goal runs out as the day goes on. I can relate this to my own personal experience. Monday morning is often 'new diet day' with a strong level of motivation. Breakfast is easy! I'm on a diet, full of energy and vigour. I take my prepared salad lunch to work. I've got this. Then comes the afternoon slump and the temptation of chocolate. The feeling is overwhelming. Motivation is running low. Do I give in or not? There lies the perennial question. The evidence is clear. Anything that requires self-control demands a lot from the 'deliberate' part of our brain and as a consequence is '*depleting and unpleasant*' (Kahneman, 2011, p 42). I eat the chocolate.

Thaler and Sunstein (2009) say that self-control is particularly difficult when choices and consequences are separated by time. Making the decision now to start writing the report due in two weeks is prone to procrastination because there is no immediate benefit. Thaler and Sunstein break down choices into 'investment goods' and 'sinful goods'. Investment goods may give limited pleasure in the short term. Taking exercise, going on a diet, flossing your teeth, or writing that report due in two weeks are possible examples. These things have limited short-term benefit but significant long-term benefit. You 'suffer' now and get the benefits later. Sinful investments like a glass of wine or a piece of cake, or finishing work early rather than doing the report give you pleasure in the short term with consequences being suffered later. Motivation is easier when we get a short-term gain and harder when the gain is in the long term. However, '*even hard problems become easier with practice*', Thaler and Sunstein tell us (2009, p 81). The more we apply ourselves to the difficult long-term goals, the easier it becomes to motivate ourselves towards them. We form a habit.

Motivation in decline

Our motivation can decline when we feel stressed and anxious with attendant physical and psychological issues that affect our productivity. There are many factors at play in terms of what drives work-related stress and anxiety, as we saw in Chapter 1. Sánchez-Moreno et al (2015) point out that social workers are an 'at risk' group when it comes to work-based stress as a consequence of the complex nature of their role and exposure to the distress they often witness. This is combined with the demands of report writing, case conferences and tight deadlines (Grant and Kinman, 2014).

Taylor (2015) makes the observation, based on empirical evidence, that a lack of resources to undertake the job undermines motivation and becomes a major barrier to accomplishing tasks. This can leave employees frustrated and feeling that their autonomy is undermined. As we have seen, autonomy plays a large role in motivation. The consequences of a lack of resources, I'm sure, are evident in many of the settings in which you work. Taylor (2015) goes on to observe that such a situation creates negativity in the workplace which in turn contributes to a less positive mindset and reduced motivation.

Motivation, and in turn productivity, also decreases as a consequence of fatigue. The longer we engage in tasks that demand our energy, the more the returns on effort invested decline. We saw in the chapter about sleep (Chapter 2) that we are biologically programmed for an afternoon sleep. It therefore comes as no surprise, given this and the fact that we will be about two thirds of the way through our working day, that productivity decreases on an afternoon. It then takes more mental effort to apply ourselves to tasks we would usually do easily (Collewet and Sauermann, 2017). Self-care has a role to play here in trying to offset some of this. As we saw in the exercise chapter, we can fuel our motivation through some gentle lunchtime exercise. We need to behave in such a way that we maximise our productivity potential by utilising the full range of self-care ideas to improve productivity. Planning to do easier, less complex tasks as motivation wanes can be helpful.

As we become fatigued and overwhelmed, our intrinsic motivation, rooted in those ideal reasons we came into the profession, gets eroded by the priority that is given to time-scales and measurable performance. When we only have so much motivation to use, we focus on the things we must do. We become motivated by extrinsic factors. It is the role of organisations and managers at all levels to create the right atmosphere so that intrinsic motivation can be left to flourish.

The calendar effect

Opinion is divided as to whether the Monday to Friday, 9 to 5, work pattern is still the best model for the workplace. Certainly, there are more flexible approaches to work these days, even when they still fit the morning to early evening, weekday format. Data is difficult to find but the European Foundation for the Improvement of Living and Working Conditions report *Changes over Time – First Findings from the Fifth European Working Conditions Survey* (2010) states that the standard five-day, 40-hour week, worked Monday to Friday, is still the norm for most Europeans. Certainly, for social workers employed in local authorities this reflects the norm although often the working hours may extend beyond 9 to 5.

This pattern dominated by the calendar is an artificial social construct that commands our attention. The calendar is an example of an external, or extrinsic, motivator, something that is external to us that motivates us to action. We've simply named the days and constructed our working life around them. Sturmey (2015) suggests that our psychological potential, and therefore our motivation, is influenced strongly by the calendar. I'm sure you will be familiar with the Sunday night blues. It's a time when 'free floating' anxiety can permeate into your world. You feel anxious but you can't attach it to anything in particular other than the fact it's the first day of work tomorrow. Then there's the Monday morning panic of checking what there is to do and figuring out how we are going to do it, and then getting over 'hump day' on a Wednesday, and then the panic rising with what's left to do before 'clocking off' on a Friday.

You can find reports of several studies on the internet (eg at Workopolis.com, 2014) that tell us something that I suspect we already instinctively know. We are at our least productive on Monday mornings and Friday afternoons and, interestingly, are at our most productive on Tuesdays. Monday mornings are often lost to planning for the week. Reacquainting ourselves with where we were up to, checking on things outstanding and planning for the week ahead. Tuesday is likely to be the most productive because we have formulated a plan on the Monday so we know what we are doing and it's early in the week so we still have some stores of energy. Once we get over the psychological 'hump day' we breathe a sigh of relief because we have done more than half the week and we are about to get some 'me time' again. Productivity starts to drop, and drops rapidly on a Friday afternoon because we get a sense that we are approaching 'our time' which lasts from late afternoon Friday to going to bed on Sunday.

Having a 'trusted system' (see 'Being organised', Chapter 7) that captures everything that there is to do in your sphere of responsibility means that you stand more chance of being able to walk away from work confident that when you return to it you will know what to do as it is all recorded there for you. This approach avoids the problem of low productivity on a Monday morning because you won't have to catch up with where you are up to and make a plan. If you had finished the week with planning, so that on Monday you already had your week organised, you could get at 'doing' much quicker. On a Friday afternoon, as your motivation wanes, you should do something constructive that will help you on Monday. What we have already seen in this chapter is that when confronted with the things we need to do we can easily be put off if things look difficult, or we don't have sufficient time, or the deadline isn't looming for us. Why do something now that will help next week? Why not just do it next week? We risk deciding to do very little as we approach 'our time' because we are, in reality, ready for a break, and that's not unreasonable. The prospect of all the wonderful things we are about to do with our weekend means we prioritise contemplating those (using our automatic brain) rather than doing something now that will help us next week. This saps our motivation. What better thing to do to energise your Friday afternoon than plan for next week! What this means is that when you finish on Friday afternoon you can leave for your weekend knowing that 'all of your ducks are in a row'. You have everything planned for next week and all the resources to hand that you will need.

I actually think that we *should* 'wind down' to our time off. But we should 'wind down' in a productive way by doing the planning I suggest. The risk of working flat out until last thing on a Friday is you go home leaving the office in a heightened state, having not planned for next week, spending the weekend at home wondering if you did everything and worrying about what there is to do next week. If you 'slide' out the week by planning to run down the pace of your work but still do things that will help you be prepared, you will have a better weekend and mitigate Sunday night anxiety.

The work–life balance myth

I've already mentioned my dislike of the concept of work–life balance in the chapter on fundamental principles (Chapter 1). I feel thinking in this way creates a binary that is often constructed as work being the thing to get out of the way, to get done, so that you can get at life. As I have previously said, work is life, and life is work, and the two have to exist together in a symbiotic relationship that enhances our productivity in all spheres and promotes a good quality of life encompassing all aspects. If you've not picked this up so far, it's worth stating – self-care is a ubiquitous lifestyle approach. It's not something you do on a weekend or on an evening. It's an approach that has to become part of you. We are trying to stay motivated in all aspects of our world. The reality that Sturmey (2015) points out is that the calendar is an enforced timetable. It's based on the idea that we give up our time Monday to Friday so that we can have our time on a weekend. The working week is a thing to be endured in order to get to the pleasure of the weekend. In reality if we are going to 'flow' then all our time needs to be enjoyed. We need to engage in self-care routinely. We need to do this throughout the week and throughout each day. We can't afford to put it to one side until the weekend or we may find ourselves too tired on a weekend to engage in any self-care at all.

Work and life should not be seen to be in competition with each other. When you're emptying the rubbish bins or stacking the dishwasher, I'm sure that feels like work rather than life. I'm sure it feels invigorating, like 'life', when you are at work and in 'flow', absorbed by a task that you delight in seeing through to completion. My personal view is that every day of your life is available to you to be in control of, as far as you can be. To be engaged in productive activity that enhances your overall life. Being autonomous and in control over what we do is a cornerstone of being motivated. We should be in charge of all of our time so that we use it all productively. 'Productive' encompasses all things. Rest, and things we can do to recuperate, are important activities that sadly we often deprioritise because they feel like a waste of time. But we should control these things and plan them. When you are at rest, sitting on the couch, binge watching *Friends*, you *are* being productive, if you have deliberately set aside time to relax and watch TV. You are actively absorbed in rest, not mindlessly absorbed in it.

Csikszentmihalyi (2002) suggests that in order to achieve flow and be deliberately involved in what we are doing we must find reward in each moment. If we gain pleasure and satisfaction from the various ongoing streams of our lives, all balanced, then '*the burden of social controls automatically falls from our shoulders*' (Csikszentmihalyi, 2002, p 19). The calendar, the demands of the workplace and the demands of our home life are no longer in control. We are in control of 'it'. 'It' isn't in control of us. Being in control, being master of our world, making autonomous decisions connected to what we are doing and who we are doing it with, is a recipe for motivation. This requires that state of 'flow' we have explored. You are engaged in the task to the exclusion of all other tasks so that nothing else seems to matter. Having a system to track things back at the office will mean you can leave it behind, enjoy your planned relaxation time and return to it refreshed and ready to engage with vigour.

PASSION AND OPTIMISM AS MOTIVATIONAL FUEL

Where is motivation rooted then and what can we do to maintain it? After all, that report is not going to write itself. We need to get started on it. We need to keep going with it. And we need to get it finished! Let's start with passion.

Pradhan et al (2017) say that passion for the work we do motivates us to seek knowledge and helps us ingrain that knowledge. We are absorbed in our profession. Purpose, they go on to say, taps us into the abundant energy that is there in us all just waiting to be discovered. Passion stimulates us to achieve goals not only at work but in all spheres of our lives. Passion can move us beyond simply bringing our cognitive, physical and emotional drivers to the practical task of work and may well lead us to see what we do as enjoyable and pleasurable (Pradhan et al, 2017). Being positive and being in a good mood promotes creativity, cognitive flexibility, innovation and responsiveness. It feels obvious to say this, but enjoying the things we do is good for us (Daisley, 2019).

Optimism is the feeling that everything is likely to turn out alright despite setbacks, problems and disappointments (Goleman, 1996). The Persian adage *'this too will pass'* is a strong mantra for me when things aren't going well, or I am feeling overwhelmed. Goleman (1996) recalls the thoughts of some of the greatest minds in this area. Martin Seligman, a renowned psychologist at the University of Pennsylvania, says that optimism is about how people explain their successes and failures to themselves. Optimists see failure as a consequence of something they could change, which could be better next time around. Pessimists see such events as outside of their control and unchangeable. Optimists respond to problems with hope and action while pessimists do nothing because, well, there's nothing they can do, is there. Albert Bandura, a psychologist at Stanford University, says that people's beliefs in their abilities have a significant impact on their actual abilities. *'People who have a sense of self-efficacy bounce back from failures; they approach things in terms of how to handle them rather than worrying about what can go wrong'* (Bandura, 1988, cited in Goleman, 1996, p 90). There's a link here to mastery that we've already looked at.

Dweck (2017) refers to this ability to see opportunities to change as having a growth mindset. She tells us that there are two sorts of people generally: those who have a fixed mindset and those who have a growth mindset. People with a fixed mindset see that their skills and abilities are fixed. They have what they have, and they are not going to get any more. People with a growth mindset see that they can use what they have to improve and develop. When a challenge presents itself they consider how they can use and develop their skills to reach the heights of skill, knowledge and ability that the task requires, rather than thinking the task is simply unachievable for 'someone like them'. This growth mindset is a great motivating force. Nelson Mandela is reported to have said, *'I never lose. I either win or learn'*. It's important not to be afraid of failure. We need to try new things to stretch ourselves, not only at work but also outside of work. I like to turn the mantra *'failure is not an option'* on its head and say that *'failure is always an option'*. We shouldn't be afraid of that. We should try a new sport, or try to cook a new recipe, or give meditation a go. If it goes wrong, we learn from it and move forward.

MOTIVATION IS IMPORTANT IN ALL ASPECTS OF OUR LIVES

I've explored motivation in this chapter largely in terms of motivating oneself at work to be productive. The same messages apply to all of the areas we think of when it comes to having a productive life and helpful self-care strategies. How we eat, exercise and sleep all rely on motivation to achieve a goal. As we have discovered, intrinsic motivators are best and such motivation is often rooted in how you set your goals. When we set goals in these areas we tend to set external goals such as being a particular weight or running a particular distance. Setting goals to be fitter, or to have more energy, or to feel good about yourself is more internally motivated and therefore more likely to be successful.

Csikszentmihalyi (2002) says that goals rooted in 'self' help us to generate a sense of purpose. When we set goals, we should make them achievable by breaking down large goals into smaller goals to make use of the psychological buzz that is achieved by the power of small wins. Having goals that draw on a sense of personal purpose should help us become immersed in the activity, be that preparing healthy food, or going for a walk, and help us to be meaningfully engaged in the activity. The sum total of these things is that we will enjoy the immediate experience. If we achieve this enjoyment, then we will be motivated to do it again. This creates flow, helps us feel in control, and helps us make sense of where the activity fits into our self-care strategy. Flow keeps us motivated.

REFERENCES

Ainslie, G (2010) Procrastination: The Basic Impulse. In Andreou, C and White, M D (eds) *The Thief of Time, Philosophical Essays on Procrastination*. New York, NY: Oxford University Press.

Allen, D (2015) *Getting Things Done: The Art of Stress-free Productivity*. London: Piatkus.

Argyris, C (1957) *Personality and Organization*. New York: Harper.

Cannon, E (2018) *Is Your Job Making You Ill?* London: Piatkus.

Cerasoli, C P, Nicklin, J M and Ford, M T (2014) Intrinsic Motivation and Extrinsic Incentives Jointly Predict Performance: A 40-year Meta-analysis. *Psychological Bulletin*, 140(4): 980–1008.

Collewet, M and Sauermann, J (2017) Working Hours and Productivity. Discussion Paper Series. IVA DP No. 10722. Bonn: IZA Institute of Labor Economics.

Coulshed, V and Mullender, A (2006) *Management in Social Work* (3rd ed). Basingstoke: Palgrave Macmillan.

Csikszentmihalyi, M (2002) *Flow*. London: Rider (The Random House Group).

Daisley, B (2019) *The Joy of Work*. London: Penguin Random House.

Dweck, C (2017) *Mindset*. London: Robinson.

European Foundation for the Improvement of Living and Working Conditions (2010) Changes Over Time: First Findings from the Fifth European Working Conditions Survey. [online] Available at: www.eurofound.europa.eu/sites/default/files/ef_files/pubdocs/2010/74/en/3/EF1074EN.pdf (accessed 4 February 2020).

Goleman, D (1996) *Emotional Intelligence: Why It Can Matter More Than IQ*. London: Bloomsbury Publishing.

Grant, L and Kinman, G (2014) What Is Resilience? In Grant, L and Kinman, G (eds) *Developing Resilience for Social Work Practice* (pp 16–30). London: Palgrave Macmillan.

Jaeger, B (2004) *Making Work Work for the Highly Sensitive Person*. New York: McGraw-Hill.

Kahneman, D (2011) *Thinking, Fast and Slow*. London: Penguin.

Levitin, D (2015) *The Organized Mind: Thinking Straight in the Age of Information Overload*. London: Penguin.

McGregor, D (1960) *The Human Side of Enterprise*. Sydney: McGraw-Hill Australia.

Newport, C (2016) *Deep Work*. London: Piatkus.

Pink, D H (2018) *Drive: The Surprising Truth about What Motivates Us*. Edinburgh: Canongate.

Pradhan, R K, Panda, P and Jena, L K (2017) Purpose, Passion, and Performance at the Workplace: Exploring the Nature, Structure, and Relationship. *The Psychologist-Manager Journal*, 20(4): 222–45.

Sánchez-Moreno, E, de La Fuente Roldán, I, Gallardo-Peralta, L P and López de Roda, A B (2015) Burnout, Informal Social Support and Psychological Distress among Social Workers. *British Journal of Social Work*, 45(8): 2368–86.

Sturmey, K (2015) *The Calendar Effect* (Kindle ed). Self-published.

Taylor, B M (2015) The Integrated Dynamics of Motivation and Performance in the Workplace. *Performance Improvement*, 54(5): 28–37.

Thaler, R H and Sunstein C R (2009) *Nudge*. London: Penguin.

Toffler, A (1970) *Futureshock*. New York: Random House.

Tracy, B (2017) *Eat That Frog*. London: Hodder and Stoughton.

Twain, M (2011) [1876] *The Adventures of Tom Sawyer* (Collins Classics). Glasgow: William Collins.

Webb, C (2017) *How to Have a Good Day: The Essential Toolkit for a Productive Day at Work and Beyond*. London: Palgrave Macmillan.

Workopolis.com (2014) *Tuesday Is the Most Productive Day of the Week*. [online] Available at: https://careers.workopolis.com/advice/tuesday-is-the-most-productive-day-of-the-week/ (accessed 4 February 2020).

Maintaining the resilient professional

Stephen

THE CHALLENGE

We all manage ourselves and our lives very differently. Remember Buckaroo? My Aunty Elva and Uncle Sid bought me the game for Christmas when I was about seven or eight years old. I loved it. The game revolves around a plastic donkey, standing firmly on all four hooves, ready to be loaded up for the day with things that need carrying. Players take turns to place items such as a shovel, a blanket and a guitar onto the donkey's back. The key thing was trying to make sure all the items loaded onto the donkey were finely balanced. Place it under too much stress and it would buck, throwing everything into disarray, scattering all of the strategically placed objects into a chaotic state. It was 'Game Over'. In order to start again you had to collect all the pieces together, reset the donkey and begin again from scratch. This is how I visualise people trying to deal with their day. They are trying to balance everything in their lives, only for it to descend into disarray. They then have to start again.

Every day we reset our donkey, collect together all of the things we need to carry, think about which ones we need to 'carry' first and then start loading them up. Unlike the game, where you only load your own things, in real life, it's worse. Other people keeping adding things to our pile of items to carry, and sometimes we don't have a choice about those things. Some of the things we want to load up never even make it onto our backs because we reach the point of 'buck'. We simply can't take any more.

Self-care and productivity are about loading things up in such a way that we don't get to the point where we buck. We have everything in its place. We are carrying what needs to be carried right now, and no more. All of the things we don't need to carry are stored safely somewhere else waiting for us to get around to doing something with them. This is your trusted system we talked about in Chapter 7 on productivity.

Another one of my favourite games growing up was Perfection. I bought the game second hand at a church fayre and loved playing it. This game was a race against the clock. With Buckaroo you had as much time as you needed to place the things on the donkey's back as carefully as possible. With this game you had a minute! You had one minute to fit all of the 26 different shapes into the right holes on a platform that was going to 'pop' upward if you didn't stop the clock before the minute was up. If you didn't succeed, the shapes would be thrown everywhere. The game started fine. It felt like you had all the time in world. As the minute got closer to being over, suddenly the game became more frantic with effortful pushing of shapes into holes that they clearly weren't meant to fit in. Then, after the minute, the spring-loaded mechanism exploded upwards sending the shapes flying everywhere, creating chaos!

I fear this is how some of us go about our days. We casually start the day by ambling in the morning, then as the day grows older, we realise we are running out of time to do everything we need to do today, so end up rushing around. If we don't get all of our shapes in their holes it all ends in disarray and we have to reorganise everything the next day to have another go at getting things done. Only now we end up having more to do! We have things from yesterday and today's things to deal with.

The more you played Perfection, the more you started to understand the game. You got to know the shapes. You got to know where they were on the playing board. You realised that by going just a little bit faster at the start, but not too fast, you didn't have to rush as much at the end. If you wanted to go 'ninja' on the game, you could line up all the similar shapes together making them more visible. I could complete the puzzle in less than a minute most of the time using this strategy.

The Buckaroo and Perfection analogies are all about how we manage what we have to do to mitigate stress. This whole book has been all about the various ways we can do just that. Our primitive stress response can be helpful, but when all of the seemingly small stresses in life are heaped one on top of each other, and our body and mind get no downtime, there can be a catastrophic effect on our health and well-being. Small stresses add up to a big mountain of stress. In the same way, small positive steps add up to big positive changes. Chatterjee (2018) calls these small stresses 'micro stress doses' and makes an interesting point about the root of many stressors being in how the world has changed. Changes have made so much of what we do a personal responsibility. Take, for example, booking a holiday. A few years back, we would have gone to a travel agent. We would have told them where we wanted to go and how much we had to spend, and they would have arranged it all for us. Now, many of us do this for ourselves and we are left with the responsibility of making sure we get it all right. It's the same with car insurance. Years ago, we went to a broker. They asked all of the questions they knew were important and got us a deal. Now we go online. We compare. We arrange our insurance and then wonder, 'Did we enter everything correctly?' 'Are the company reputable?' 'Did I enter everything I should?'

It's the same in the workplace. Many processes have administrative functions that have now been reallocated to practitioners, thus increasing their workload and leaving them thinking more about getting those things right than about their actual face-to-face practice.

You are only one person, or, like in Buckaroo, one donkey. You can only carry so much 'stuff' before you will have had enough. How carefully you load that stuff up is crucial. You will be able to carry stuff more effectively if you load it up sensibly. You will be able to carry it for long enough to deal with it, freeing up time to do other self-care things. If you work long hours, it's harder to find the time to self-care. Not impossible, but harder. There comes a point where you must prioritise yourself.

Even if you do all of the things in this book, and I urge you to, you may find that you are still being asked to do too much. It's **your** professional responsibility to raise this with your manager. This is not just the case at work. At home you need to think in the same way. Are you being asked to do too much by family and friends? Again, if you have used the advice in this book, and you are still overwhelmed, then maybe you need to have a 'supervision' session with your friends and family. You are only one person.

Having a trusted system will help you organise all of the things you need to do, all of those shapes that need to fit into the correct hole, much more effectively. Not perfectly, because life isn't perfect, and sometimes you won't get everything done in the time you have. But if, more often than not, you manage to press stop on the clock before everything explodes, then you will have kept everything in its correct place. If the worst happens and there is a crisis, you will find it easier to put all of the shapes back if you are skilled at putting the shapes in the holes in the first place.

The ideas we've presented take time to get up and running. It took me about three months of tinkering with my trusted system until I was happy I had everything in it. Most of it was done quite quickly but things kept popping up that I had to add in. Getting everything done to keep things from 'popping up' is about being consistent in your approach. More often than not it allows the stop button to be pressed before chaos ensues. Then you can take time out for 'me' and return to dealing with any new shapes when rested. Plan first, then do. Group your tasks together into groups of similar tasks.

THE HIGHLY SENSITIVE PERSON

In the summer of 2019, while on holiday, driving back to our rented cottage in North Yorkshire, I stumbled across a Radio 4 show *Hannah Walker Is a Highly Sensitive Person* (BBC Sounds, 2019) that sparked an idea worthy of some significant investigation. Hannah Walker, a poet and theatre maker, was talking with a psychologist and a neuroscientist about the idea of the 'highly sensitive person'. Hannah, who states she is a highly sensitive person herself, was talking about how sensitivity is often overlooked, dismissed and seen as a weakness. One of her guests told her a story about how, as a teacher, she was overworking so as not to fail her pupils. In doing so, she said, she actually was failing them, as she was so tired when at work, preventing her from giving her best. She didn't blame the particular school, but rather the way people are asked, or choose, to work that results in them deciding to leave their chosen profession. This is a familiar story to us in social work.

Hannah also interviewed an academic who talked of research that showed we all perceive, process and respond to our environments differently, yet work settings presume everyone is the same. The academic described how highly sensitive people respond to the emotions of others differently as the reward centres in their brains are more activated than is usual when reacting to the emotions of others. During another interview, a computer software consultant talked about how his industry was using highly sensitive people to explore the user experience of computer programs, as they are better at listening, picking up on people's body language and engaging people by asking them '*What would you expect instead?*' when they recognise something clearly isn't working for the user. Does that sound familiar to you as a social worker?

Her final guest talked about the professions where people may experience secondary trauma: people in medicine, the police and ... social work. Highly sensitive people are attrantr·l tu tñc̠ᴄ̠ᴇ̠ prōfessions as they have the right skill set for such roles. They show more empathetic concern and more emotional intelligence, but this comes at the cost of increased emotional distress. So, if social work attracts highly sensitive people, then surely what this means is that self-care is more important than it would be for people who are not highly sensitive. If a certain profession attracts a particular 'type' of person then surely the work culture of that profession needs to be tailored to their nature. There is a role here for self-care initiated both by oneself and by organisations to offer support to promote well-being. It needs people to have trusted systems for being organised so they can engage more effectively in the work they are 'designed' for without it making them ill.

In the late 1990s Aron and Aron developed a method for assessing if someone was a highly sensitive person, hypothesising that this innate ability was measurable (Smith et al, 2019). This is worthy, I feel, of some research inquiry. Anecdotally, in conversations with practising social workers and social work students, they relate both to the term highly sensitive person and to the traits that Aron and Aron identify as likely indicators. The idea they readily 'take on' the emotions of others, often at the expense of their own, has resonance. Stories of stress, overwhelm, burnout and compassion fatigue attest to the urgency of some serious exploration in this area.

Highly sensitive people are likely to see their response to the emotional content of their labours as negative. They feel they are somehow failing because they respond emotionally and not pragmatically. The reality is we probably need a balance of these two things. When they feel negative, the already intense stress is amplified and feelings of hopelessness and worthlessness overwhelm (Aron, 1999). The reality is that good social work is about what highly sensitive people are good at: understanding, reading and reacting to people's emotions. That 'cost' needs to be somehow managed. Counselling literature talks about creating a safe space. That 'safe space' could be a location or an individual. Whatever it is it needs to be something. It could be your manager in supervision, it could be a friend or colleague who understands you, or it could be under a tree in the park with a cappuccino. There should be both a formal and an informal space for this.

Think about the 'safe spaces' you can create. These may be at work or at home. They may be people or places or things to do. Where do you 'go', physically and metaphorically, to feel safe and to explore your emotions?

What is it that distresses you to the point where you need to seek out a 'safe space'?

Do you find you don't seek out 'safe spaces' when you should? Could you do more to seek out 'safe spaces' at times of crisis? What could you plan to do?

Could you be more self-disciplined in using your safe spaces? Could you carve out time to spend in your safe spaces? Could you plan 'safe space' time in advance creating a time-out zone?

(Created with Jaeger, 2004, p 73 in mind)

THE IMPACT OF WHERE YOU ARE

Responsibility for self-care lies both in the individual and in the organisation they work in. There is a responsibility to ensure manageable workloads and good quality reflective supervision. You have a responsibility to bring problems in these areas to the attention of your manager and your organisation. I fear that at times we become complicit because we stop raising our voices. Continuing to work beyond your capacity, or, as a manager, accepting your team are working beyond their capacity, is detrimental not only to the individuals but also ultimately to the organisation's reputation. It is equally, and alarmingly, detrimental to the very vulnerable people we are employed to serve. Egbert Cadbury (of the chocolate makers) said '*Business efficiency and the welfare of employees are but two sides of the same problem*' (Rose, 1999, p 61). This is not an easy conundrum to solve. I am not in the business of hostility towards managers and senior managers, as they are also labouring in a system undermined by political ideology and austerity, but we can't simply accept this as the way it is. We all must continue to 'push back' and not accept that this is the only way it can be. Our protest needs to be constructive, not hostile. Sadly, I often see the latter.

THE CONTEMPORARY OFFICE ENVIRONMENT

It seems hot-desking and agile working is now the norm. Opinion is divided on whether these concepts are helpful. The key is to think about how we turn this to our advantage as practitioners. What is it about hot-desking and being 'agile' that could improve our productivity and what is it that gets in the way? Where we work, as well as how we work, can have an impact. Daisley (2019) states working at home can offer peace and tranquillity and can be a real positive for people who need to balance home and work commitments. But it is in the flow of ideas where he sees a downside. Teams who work together, he says, create a collective intelligence. This is true of social work teams. I tell students all of the time, '*Keep asking questions, everyone else does, even those who are experienced.*' They report back to me this is indeed true. They hear social workers checking things out with each other and debating the value of different approaches to complex situations. Daisley (2019) also notes that while home working in a tranquil environment gives an initial productivity boost this can soon dissipate because of the lack of connection.

On the other hand, Newport (2016) argues that at times we need to engage in what he terms 'deep work'. This is work that requires contemplation, concentration and reflection. Such work needs peace and quiet to consider things that we can't resolve quickly and that need careful thought. The things that need long periods of concentration are simply not suitable for an open plan, hot-desking, environment.

HOT-DESKING

Jeyasingham's research (2016) suggests while the move to hot-desking is often about the financial implications of expensive office space, it also offers the opportunity to base relationships on trust rather than hierarchy. We've seen that autonomy offers significant opportunities to promote well-being and achieve a state of flow, and agile working seems to offer that. He suggests the literature on the subject says agile working brings people and process into the same space and allows for a more responsive way of working, but also notes that the office space is good for reflection, discussion and support from colleagues. Jeyasingham conducted research in 2019 to explore how a team of children's social workers were using agile working. He found people tended to homework when they had in-depth pieces of work to complete, like court reports, because they valued the solitude and the quiet environment. The participants reported they could be more immersed in their work and this came from the comfort of being at home and being able to moderate extraneous noise. While it was flexible and convenient, people also reported they worked longer hours (Jeyasingham, 2019). This is a risk with agile working, that you never switch off and the temptation is always there to check emails late on an evening or at the weekend. You need to monitor and manage this. It takes self-discipline.

I personally find it helpful to spend an hour on a Sunday afternoon checking my work emails as I find that I enjoy my evening more knowing what is in store on Monday morning. The fear of what is there can sometimes be worse than what is actually there. Even when there is something concerning there, I can formulate a plan, put it in my calendar and know that it's the first thing I will get onto when I'm at work. I can count on one hand the number of times this strategy has caused me a sleepless night. This may not be the strategy for you, but I describe it to show the highly personal nature of our relationship with getting things done. It is essential you find what works specifically for you.

Despite our views on whether agile working and hot-desking are good things or bad things, I hazard a guess that for the foreseeable future they are here to stay. Even with the problems they bring they do bring positives. We need to find what those positives are for us. Newport (2016) suggests that the secret to successful productivity is to place yourself in the best location to do the thing you most need to do at that point in time. If that is deep work, then you need a quiet space without interruption. If you need a stimulating environment that keeps you motoring through tasks, then that could be a coffee shop. Jeyasingham (2019) reported that social workers in the study he conducted found coffee shops suitable for responding to emails and writing certain types of reports. There are obvious concerns about confidentiality but, as someone who works in coffee shops quite a bit, I can say that these things are not insurmountable. In the study people said they positioned themselves in a quiet part of the cafe or with a wall behind them, so they weren't overlooked. (For my work laptop I have been provided with a privacy screen overlay that means the screen is not visible unless you are directly in front of it.) The participants in the study even noted that between visits the car was a good place to make phone calls, maximising what they did in the time they had. These ideas require you to be organised with everything you need to hand. It would help to plan and 'chunk' tasks together (see Chapter 7 on productivity) so you are ready to do the appropriate tasks in the appropriate places.

You may also choose to place yourself in a communal environment, like the hot-desking team room, when you need to exchange ideas or think things through. You can seek out your colleagues and thrash out a difficult issue. Daisley (2019) says that when creativity is required, being around others is stimulating. When you are hot-desking you may find yourself sitting with people who you wouldn't normally sit with. This can stimulate thinking and lead to the cross fertilisation of ideas. Social work is an art not a science and art needs creative thinking.

THINK ABOUT THE ADVANTAGES OF THE PLACES YOU WORK

- Consider a time when you were completely absorbed in something, when you were in the 'flow'. What was your environment like? What was the task you were undertaking? Note this for future reference as a place conducive to doing that task.
- Think about times you get nothing done because you are distracted. Where are you? What distracts you? How could you minimise the distractions?
- For managers, think about the areas of work where you can give your staff more autonomy. Think about whether you can be more flexible with where, when and how your staff work.

THE 'THRIVE' STATE

Maintaining your well-being is a complex mix of who you are, where you are doing what you are doing, how well you eat, sleep and exercise, and how organised you are. All of these things need your attention to some degree or other. How much you need to consider each element depends on who you are and what you are doing but I guarantee you need to consider all of these to some degree. We all need a unique self-care balance which we can only find through experimentation. Chatterjee (2018) points out that to your body, everything is information. Your senses explore the environment, your guts explore what you eat, and your immune system checks on what is happening physically and emotionally. He suggests that how you manage all of these areas influences whether your body places itself into a stress state or a 'thrive' state. We are trying to achieve a thrive state. To do this you need to understand yourself. The best social workers, I tell students, are the ones that know themselves the best. They understand how they respond emotionally, they can acknowledge when they are fatigued before it's too late, and they know how to return to their self-care strategies if they've lost their way. The thrive state relies on how well you sleep, your nutrition and how physically prepared you have made your body through exercise. All of these things, as we've seen, influence your mental and emotional health, and those things affect how productive you are.

MAINTAINING ENERGY

Being in a 'thrive' state creates energy but how do you keep your energy topped up?

Think of three good, positive things that have happened to you (sometimes referred to as a gratitude exercise). Write them down. Do this every day or when you need a boost.

Engage in a random act of kindness. Just be nice to someone.

Find something interesting. I have lots of books dotted around the place that have little snippets or slogans within them that I can just pick up and read for a minute or so. Take time out to look at a painting or read a poem.

Give yourself a quick win. Finding it difficult to motivate yourself? Find something that you can get done quickly. Use the two-minute rule from Chapter 7.

Go and talk to someone. Getting nowhere? Get up from your desk and say, '*Anyone want a coffee?*' Or walk out of the office and chat to whoever you see first.

Sit quietly and breathe in for three, hold for three and breathe out for three. Do this as many times as you want.

Drink a glass of water.

Go for a quick walk outside and breathe deeply.

Smile. Smiling is contagious. Smile at someone and they generally smile back, but more than that, smiling creates a mind–body loop that makes you feel happy. Try it.

Adapted from Webb (2017)

VISUALISATION

We are products of our thoughts. Our actions are products of our thoughts. You will no doubt have watched many sportsmen and -women visualising what they are about to do. They visualise the rugby ball going in between the posts from the penalty kick or they rehearse the golf swing before teeing off. In a Harvard experiment researchers took two groups of people and taught both groups to play a sequence of notes on the piano. They then asked them to practise for a week so they could test their accuracy throughout the week. One group could actually play the notes on the keyboard while the other group had to sit at the keyboard and simply visualise themselves playing the notes. On the third day of the experiment both groups were equally as accurate. The group with physical access to the keyboard had started to edge ahead by day five but only one session on the actual keyboard caught the other group up. Mind's-eye rehearsal works. It fires the same parts of your brain as actually undertaking the task physically does, activating neural connections (Webb, 2017). Tracy (2017) comments that people who visualise their goals generate focus and energy. They feel a greater sense of control and personal power.

Visualisation requires a plan. You need to know what you are going to visualise. When you leave the house to go on a trip you don't climb into the car and say, *'let's go'* and drive off, taking random left or right turns and just ending up somewhere (unless of course you are on a mystery tour!). This is how lots of people live their lives day to day, week to week, year to year. When you go on a road trip it is more likely that you will have already planned where to go. You will have figured out a route. You may have checked the weather to see if the activity you will do when you arrive is possible. If it's a long journey you will have definitely bought travelling sweets. If you don't know where you are going you won't know how to get there and you won't know what to visualise.

Have you got a plan? Have you got a ten-year plan? What are you aiming for? Have you got a plan for next year? Have you got a plan for next week? Without a plan how do you know what to do? I left my job in IT to train to be a social worker. I enrolled on a programme and found myself sitting in my first sociology lecture. I watched the lecturer do her stuff and I was in awe. I thought, *'That's what I want to do, that there!'* My ten-year plan was set in motion. Everything I then did centred around that ten-year plan. I put myself forward for training, I fed things back at team meetings to overcome my dreadful shyness, I trained to be a 'practice educator' to keep theory in my head, and I volunteered to go into the local university to do practitioner-led sessions. Twelve years later, so a little behind schedule, I landed a job as a lecturer. When I turned 50, I created my ten-year plan to carry me through to 60. By the time I'm 60 I want my work to be completely freelance. When I started creating that plan I had no idea what I'd do as a freelancer, only some vague notions on writing and lecturing. I just knew I didn't want to work for someone else. I wanted to work for myself doing what I wanted to do, when I wanted to do it. I created my social work blog, I began to talk to people about teaching self-care and productivity, and through a chance connection I was offered a contract to write for an education provider – and now, here I am writing a book. That's just two years into my ten-year plan. If you know where you want to go you start making decisions that work towards that objective. You visualise yourself where you want to be.

This works just as well for what you might be doing next week or even tomorrow. On a daily basis go to your diary and visualise doing the tasks you find in there with great aplomb to a successful conclusion, then visualise yourself relaxing at the end of the day after being productive and completely in control. What will you have achieved? How will you feel? Work through each thing you will do. 'Watch' yourself doing it well and getting it done. Feel the delight of having achieved. Use all of your senses. Create the image of what tomorrow will look like and how you will feel at the end of it. *'Who we are and where we want to go determine what we do and what we accomplish'* (Keller and Papasan, 2014, p 139). Visualise it, then do it. Most of what we have talked about in this book demands you focus on single tasks one at a time to the exclusion of everything else. Visualisation and creating the 'big picture' plan is your chance to let your senses run wild and think about it all. Meaning and purpose, Chatterjee (2018) says, are the things missing from the lives of most. *'Filling your life with meaning and purpose is the single most important thing you can do to live the life you've always dreamed of'* (Chatterjee, 2018, p 26).

THE IMPORTANCE OF ROUTINE

The internet is awash with stories about productive people and I want to share some of them with you. One of the common themes is routine. Routine creates order. It creates a sense of knowing where you are, and the right sort of routines can place the right things in the right place at the right time. I can't verify the accuracy of these routines, but the stories of how people structure their days show us how some of the ideas we have presented can be integrated into daily life. They are from a blog at thoughtcatalog.com (Thought Catalog, 2019), with inserted comments (italics).

Benjamin Franklin (American Founding Father, died 1790)

4am: Wake, wash, eat breakfast, and think about what I want to accomplish for the day.

This is an early start and only affords him six hours sleep. The research we've seen suggests sleeping a little longer. What this does show though is a routine start to the day and visualisation of what he wants to achieve. This looks like it is his planning stage before getting on to the doing.

8am–12pm: Work.

He has a clear time slot for work. He has planned earlier and now gets on to doing.

12pm–1pm: Lunch while reading or looking over accounts.

He breaks for lunch. He's looking over accounts, and while it's better to eat lunch without 'doing', he's at least changed what he's been doing to something different. 'Chunking' in action maybe?

1pm–5pm: Work.

5pm: Conclude work, finish the day with dinner, putting things in their place, music and conversation, and reflect on the day.

He has a routine for his evening that includes time for himself, time to socialise and time to reflect. Reflection can often lead into meditation and mindfulness.

10pm: Bed.

This bedtime is perfect given what we found out in the sleep chapter.

Henry Miller (American writer, died 1980)

Mornings: If groggy, type notes and allocate as stimulus. If in 'fine fettle', write.

This shows Miller's understanding of his chronotype. He knows he is not going to be on top form every morning, so he has a plan to still be productive. He types notes to create stimulus. He understands what will motivate him.

Afternoons: Write to finish one section at a time, for good and all.

He understands the importance of breaking the task down into sections so that you can get a section done and feel the benefit of the power of small wins.

Evenings: See friends. Read in cafes. Explore unfamiliar sections – on foot if wet, on bicycle if dry. Write, if in mood, but only on Minor programme. Paint if empty or tired. Make notes, charts, plans, corrections.

He understands the importance of time to himself and time with his friends. He has something he goes to when he feels tired – painting. Painting can be a therapeutic activity. You can get lost in such a craft and it is a form of mindfulness or meditation. He also gets some exercise walking or cycling.

Barack Obama (President of the United States, 2009–17)

6.45am: Work out, read several newspapers, have breakfast with family.

8.50am: Begin work just before 9.

10pm: Work well into many evenings, but always stop to have dinner with family each day.

Obama's routine is very simple and is very work focused, probably because he was the president at the time. But it has some important things in there. It has exercise built in daily to launch the day and it has family time at the start and at the end. Our connection to people is very important for our well-being and therefore our productivity.

Charles Darwin (naturalist, geologist and biologist, died 1882)

I particularly like this routine, which was found on the When I Work blog (wheniwork. com, 2019).

7am: Wake up and take a short walk.

This is a great start to the day. The perfect time to wake up, and a walk outside is a great way to start the day. Being outside in morning sunlight starts processes that can lead to a good night's sleep.

7.45am: Breakfast alone

This may well have provided a time of quiet reflection which is a type of mindfulness or meditation.

8–9.30am: Work in study.

This is a good focused 'chunk' of work. The modern work ethic says we start and then we keep going without a break. What we know is that intense periods of work, where we have chunked similar tasks together, is a good way to work. But we can only stay focused and motivated for so long before we need to recharge. That can be by taking time out or changing the type of task. An hour and a half is probably manageable for most.

9.30–10.30am: On to the drawing-room and read letters, followed by reading aloud of family letters.

Here he has chunked tasks together. Reading general letters and family letters, and the family letters are read aloud so that it provides time with his family to hear from others.

10.30am–12pm: Walk (alone or with dog).

More thinking and reflective time. I find walking my dog a great opportunity to switch off and take time out. I just watch the dog running around or sniffing about and try to forget everything else. If thoughts pop into my head I decide to entertain them and try and work through whatever the issue might be, or I dismiss them until another time, sometimes making a note in my smartphone.

12pm: Return to study.

Fully recharged Darwin gets back to work.

3pm: Resting in bedroom on the sofa and smoking a cigarette *(not recommended!)* and listening to a novel or other light literature read by my wife Emma.

What a great way to spend the afternoon! The modern equivalent is probably the audio book. But either way this is more downtime. Darwin's routine shows clearly that he has time for serious thinking and work as well as time for relaxation and recuperation. Having a break at this time fits with our biological need for a snooze in the afternoon.

4pm: Walk.

The importance of exercise is clearly understood by Darwin. He will come back with a clear head, recharged and ready to start again with the next task.

4.30–5.30pm: Work in study, clearing up daily matters.

This period of time looks like a chance to get things finished so if it can be done it doesn't hang around until the next day. It feels like a chance to complete things and then plan for tomorrow.

6pm: Resting again, with Emma reading aloud.

Having someone read to you, I imagine, is quite therapeutic. You can absorb yourself in the text and the voice to the exclusion of other things, again offering an opportunity for mindful attention.

7pm: Tea, reading and games.

More downtime! I don't think in this modern world we could achieve quite this level of leisure activity but maybe we should. This part of the day seems to be spent with others to play games which is excellent for our well-being.

10pm: Left the drawing-room and usually in bed by 10.30pm.

This is the perfect time to go to bed. He clearly has a routine to prepare for bed as it takes him half an hour.

What you will see here is that all of these routines are different. Some are complex, some quite simple. By having a routine these people can fit into their lives what they need to fit in. Repetition of a routine creates a habit and habits mean we automate our 'getting things done'. Habits create flow. Flow creates momentum and focus. Momentum motivates and focus helps us to get on with things.

LET'S GO BACK TO WHERE WE STARTED

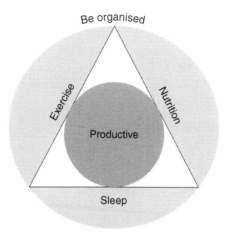

Productivity is at the heart of successful lives. Productivity is not just about work lives. It is about whole lives. We need to be productive in our family life, our work life, our life with friends and our life as part of a community, or many communities. Being productive makes us feel good and feeling good makes us more productive.

Some things are outside of our control, but many things are within our reach to grasp. Productivity is surrounded by the triangle of sleep, exercise and nutrition. While we have explored these elements as separate chapters, they are all intertwined. Sleep is the cornerstone. Get that right first. Then think about being active and think about what you eat. All of these things have an impact on our productivity, largely because of the impact they have, positive or negative, on how we feel. We must therefore understand our emotions. The emotional content of our lives is influenced by these three things and, in turn, influences how we approach them. Goleman (1996) talks about being competent pilots of our lives. Rather than having our emotions swamp us we need to manage them skilfully. That can only come through understanding ourselves. Understanding ourselves comes from self-reflection and self-reflection means spending time away from distractions in a mindful or meditative state. Know yourself.

Surrounding all of this is being organised. If you don't structure your day, your week, your month, your year and your life, you will be leaving a great deal to chance. For some that has a great appeal, and I understand that. *'Let's just see what tomorrow brings'*. For me, I have this one chance at this life, and I want to make every part of it count. If you haven't got a plan, then how do you know where you are going?

Make a plan.

Engage with your plan.

Live your life.

Be productive.

REFERENCES

Aron, E N (1999) *The Highly Sensitive Person.* Croydon: Harper Collins.

BBC Sounds (2019) Hannah Walker Is a Sensitive Person. Radio programme. [online] Available at: www.bbc.co.uk/sounds/play/m0007bkj (accessed 25 February 2020).

Chatterjee, R (2018) *The Stress Solution.* London: Penguin.

Daisley, B (2019) *The Joy of Work.* London: Penguin Random House.

Goleman, D (1996) *Emotional Intelligence: Why It Can Matter More Than IQ.* London: Bloomsbury Publishing.

Jaeger, B (2004) *Making Work Work for the Highly Sensitive Person.* New York, NY: McGraw-Hill.

Jeyasingham, D (2016) Open Spaces, Supple Bodies? Considering the Impact of Agile Working on Social Work Office Practices. *Child and Family Social Work,* 21(2): 209–17.

Jeyasingham, D (2019) Seeking Solitude and Distance from Others: Children's Social Workers' Agile Working Practices and Experiences beyond the Office. *British Journal of Social Work,* 49(3): 559–76.

Keller, G and Papasan, J (2014) *The One Thing.* London: John Murray.

Newport, C (2016) *Deep Work.* London: Piatkus.

Rose, N (1999) *Governing of the Soul: The Shaping of the Private Self* (2nd ed). London: Free Association Books.

Smith, H L, Sriken, J and Bradley T E (2019) Clinical and Research Utility of the Highly Sensitive Person Scale. *Journal of Mental Health Counseling,* 41(3): 221–41.

Thought Catalog (2019) 12 Daily Routines of Famous People in History – And What You Should Take from Each. [online] Available at: https://thoughtcatalog.com/brianna-wiest/2015/11/12-daily-routines-of-famous-people-in-history-and-what-you-should-take-from-each/ (accessed 4 February 2020).

Tracy, B (2017) *Eat That Frog.* London: Hodder and Stoughton.

Webb, C (2017) *How to Have a Good Day: The Essential Toolkit for a Productive Day at Work and Beyond.* London: Palgrave Macmillan.

Wheniwork.com (2019) Famous People's Schedules. [online] Available at: https://wheniwork.com/blog/famous-people-schedules-infographic/ (accessed 4 February 2020).

INDEX